Pocket Reference to

Cytomegalovirus Infection

Contents

Author biography

Vincent C Emery is currently Professor of Virology at University College London (UCL) and also Pro-Provost (South Asia and the Middle East). Professor Emery started his academic career graduating with a 1st-class BSc (Hons) in Biochemistry and Chemistry from the University of Southampton, UK. He then worked under the auspices of Professor Muhammad Akhtar FRS at Southampton University to complete his PhD in 1985 in mechanistic biochemistry. His interests in molecular virology were first cultivated when he undertook a 3-year postdoctoral fellowship working with Professor David Bishop at the then NERC Institute of Virology, Oxford. During this time he worked on a number of exotic virus infections, including Rift Valley fever virus and Punta Toro virus, before developing the first multiple baculovirus expression system that enabled the high-level production of two proteins simultaneously. These vectors and their successors have been extensively used throughout the world to investigate multiprotein complexes and virus assembly. Professor Emery took up a Lectureship in Molecular Virology at the Royal Free Hospital School of Medicine in 1988 (now a part of the Royal Free and University College Medical School of UCL). During the past 18 years his research has focused on viruses of medical importance, including the beta-herpesviruses, especially cytomegalovirus. Using a combination of molecular, virological, mathematical, biological and, more recently, immunological approaches his research aims to provide a holistic approach to understanding why cytomegalovirus causes disease and how antiviral therapy can be deployed to prevent disease in the immunocompromised host. Professor Emery's research group have made a number of seminal discoveries in the field of cytomegalovirus research, including defining the central role that viral replication and viral load plays in pathogenesis and the fact that cytomegalovirus replication is highly dynamic with doubling times as quick as 1 day.

Abbreviations

AIDS	acquired immune deficiency syndrome
BAL	bronchoalveolar lavage
BLQ	below the level of quantitation
BTS	British Transplantation Society
CI	confidence interval
CMV	cytomegalovirus
CNS	central nervous system
CSF	cerebrospinal fluid
D	donor
DNA pol	DNA polymerase
E	early
EBV	Epstein–Barr virus
ELISA	enzyme-linked immunosorbent assay
gB	glycoprotein B
gH	glycoprotein H
GCV	ganciclovir
GVHD	graft-versus-host disease
HAART	highly active antiretroviral therapy
HCMV	human cytomegalovirus
HHV	human herpes virus
HIV	human immunodeficiency virus
HLA	human leukocyte antigen
HSCT	haematopoietic stem cell transplant
HSV	herpes simplex virus
ICAM-1	intercellular adhesion molecule
IE	immediate early
IFN	interferon
Ig	immunoglobulin
IHMF	International Herpes Management Forum
IV	intravenous
L	late
LFA	lymphocyte function-associated antigen 1
MHC	major histocompatibility complex
MP	monophosphate
mRNA	messenger ribonucleic acid
NF-κB	nuclear factor-κB
NK	natural killer

PCR	polymerase chain reaction
RCT	randomised controlled trial
SNHL	sensorineural hearing loss
SOT	solid organ transplant
TK	thymidine kinase
TNF	tumour necrosis factor
TP	triphosphate
VCAM	vascular cell adhesion molecule
VLA	very late antigen
VZV	varicella-zoster virus

1

Introduction

Human cytomegalovirus (HCMV; *see* Figure 1.1) is a member of the *Herpesviridae*, together with other notable human viral agents such as herpes simplex virus types 1 and 2, varicella-zoster virus and Epstein–Barr virus (*see* Table 1.1). Of these, HCMV has the largest genome, with a 236-kb double-stranded DNA [1,2]. Herpes viruses are widespread in the general population and are characterised by their ability to remain dormant in the body over a long period following the initial infection. As such, herpes viruses give rise to persistent and latent forms of infection. HCMV, designated human herpes virus 5 (HHV-5) in the systematic nomenclature, is a member of the *Betaherpesvirinae* subfamily, along with two more recently characterised herpes viruses, HHV-6 and HHV-7 (*see* Table 1.1). HCMV is characterised by its restricted host range (it replicates only in human cells), the production of inclusion bodies (cytomegalia), and a long replication cycle *in vitro* [3].

HCMV is found universally throughout all geographical locations and socioeconomic groups. In developed countries, up to three-quarters of the adult population are seropositive for HCMV –

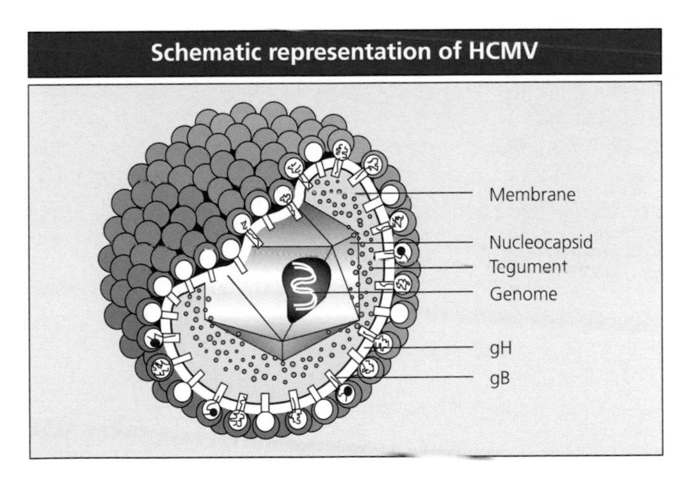

Figure 1.1

Classification of the human herpes viruses		
Human herpes virus	**Abbreviation**	**Classification**
Herpes simplex virus 1	HSV-1	alpha (α)
Herpes simplex virus 2	HSV-2	alpha (α)
Varicella-zoster virus	VZV	alpha (α)
Cytomegalovirus	HCMV	beta (β)
Human herpes virus 6	HHV-6	beta (β)
Human herpes virus 7	HHV-7	beta (β)
Epstein–Barr virus	EBV	gamma (γ)
Human herpes virus 8 (Kaposi's sarcoma-associated herpes virus)	HHV-8	gamma (γ)

Table 1.1.

seropositivity in the absence of replicating virus indicates the presence of latent virus that may be reactivated to cause clinical disease. In contrast, in developing countries and areas of low socioeconomic status, HCMV seroprevalence may be as high as 90–100%. HCMV infection is mostly acquired during early childhood, with viral transmission occurring in up to 80% of infants in day-care centres and around 20% of children cared for in the home [4]. The prevalence of infection increases with age after infancy. About 40–80% of adolescents are infected, while beyond adolescence, the rate of infection increases by around 1% per year. Therefore, HCMV has been estimated to infect between 60% and 90% of healthy individuals [5].

Transmission of HCMV usually occurs from person to person. HCMV is a relatively unstable virus and its horizontal transmission requires direct contact with bodily secretions that contain the virus. HCMV may be shed in the bodily fluids of any previously infected person and can be found in urine, saliva, blood, tears, semen and breast milk. Routes of transmission of HCMV include:

- intrauterine, which causes congenital infection due to maternal viraemia during pregnancy;

- perinatal, due to contact of the infant with infected maternal genital secretions during birth and/or through breast milk; and
- horizontal transmission (direct and indirect contact).

It is widely believed that sexual contact (oral and/or genital) is one of the main modes of transmission in adults. Horizontal transmission of HCMV may often be preventable through attention to personal hygiene; for example, hand washing with soap and water to remove the virus from the hands.

Solid organ or stem cell transplantation can also lead to transmission of HCMV, with the risk of infection depending on the serological status of the transplant donor and recipient. Approximately 75% of solid organ transplant recipients have some evidence of active HCMV infection (ie, evidence of viral replication in blood using methods such as cell culture, antigenaemia and the polymerase chain reaction [PCR]) in the first 3 months following transplant in the absence of antiviral prophylaxis for HCMV [6]. The highest risk of severe HCMV disease in solid organ transplantation occurs with the seropositive donor–seronegative recipient (D^+R^-) combination [7]. When both donor and recipient are seropositive (D^+R^+), the recipient may reactivate their own virus or be reinfected by the donor HCMV strain. In these patients, there is an intermediate risk of severe disease compared with the high-risk D^+R^- category. The lowest risk of HCMV disease occurs in the seronegative donor–seronegative recipient (D^-R^-) setting, provided these patients receive HCMV-negative blood or leukodepleted blood products. Other risk factors for the development of HCMV disease in solid organ transplant recipients include the level of immunosuppression in the recipient, their age, comorbidity and any co-infection, the use of induction or anti-rejection therapy, and the type of transplant. Heart, heart–lung, lung, small intestine and pancreas transplant recipients are considered to be at the highest risk for HCMV disease, whereas liver and kidney recipients are at a slightly lower risk [4].

In stem cell transplantation, the highest risk of HCMV disease occurs when a seropositive recipient receives donor cells from a seronegative donor, since the reactivation of endogenous HCMV within the recipient occurs in the context of a regenerating immune system that has not previously encountered HCMV.

HCMV disease can be particularly problematic in patients receiving T-cell-depleted transplants to decrease the incidence of graft-versus-host disease. Similar to the situation described above in solid organ transplantation, when both donor and recipient are seropositive, re-infection and reactivation may occur.

Transmission of HCMV through blood transfusion is now extremely rare, even when the donor is seropositive and the recipient is seronegative for the virus.

Three major epidemiological patterns of HCMV infection (*see* Table 1.2) are observed:

- primary infection;
- reactivation or secondary infection; and
- superinfection or re-infection.

As mentioned earlier, HCMV is an opportunistic virus that remains latent in the body following primary infection. Although the sites of latency have not been fully elucidated, bone marrow progenitor cells and cells of monocytic origin are prime candidates. Nevertheless, other sites of latency may also be important.

HCMV can cause a variety of clinical syndromes, including cytomegalic inclusion disease in the neonate and, occasionally, hepatitis and a mononucleosis-like syndrome during primary infection of the immunocompetent host. However, in most healthy, immunocompetent individuals, HCMV acquired after birth is associated with few, if any, symptoms and no long-term health consequences. After primary infection, the virus establishes lifelong latency through relatively poorly defined mechanisms. Long-term immunity involving the production of a broad-spectrum antibody response, including neutralising antibodies directed towards the viral envelope glycoproteins and a wide-spectrum CD4 and CD8 T-cell response, is established after this initial infection and appears to suppress viral replication in the immunocompetent host. Thus, periodic reactivations in the immunocompetent host probably do not result in extensive replication and rarely, if ever, result in symptoms [3]. Although, the direct effects of HCMV infection do not appear to be a major issue in the immunocompetent host, HCMV seropositivity has been associated with a number of so-called indirect effects involving

Epidemiological patterns of HCMV infection
Primary infection
Initial infection with HCMV in a seronegative individual • Congenital HCMV infection is mainly related to primary maternal infection [8] • In the solid organ transplant setting, primary infection occurs when an HCMV-seronegative individual receives an allograft from an HCMV-seropositive donor with the transfer of latently infected cells occurring during transplantation [6] – the incidence of symptomatic HCMV infection in seronegative recipients of allografts from seropositive donors is 50–65% [6]
Reactivation or secondary infection
Reactivation of endogenous latent HCMV in a seropositive individual • In the transplant setting, episodes of reactivation occur when a seropositive recipient of an allograft reactivates their endogenous virus derived from latently infected cells within the organs of the host [6] – the incidence of symptomatic HCMV infection in seropositive recipients of allografts from seropositive donors is 15–20% [6] • Reactivation appears to be less common for HCMV than for other herpes viruses, such as Epstein–Barr virus and herpes simplex virus • Specific stimuli are required to initiate the HCMV replicative cycle, with TNF-α acting as a key mediator of reactivation
Superinfection or re-infection
Re-infection of a seropositive individual by a new strain of HCMV • In the transplant setting, superinfection or re-infection occurs when a seropositive recipient receives an allograft from a seropositive donor and reactivation of latent virus occurs in the allograft (ie, the virus that is reactivated is of donor origin) [6] • Superinfection may occur in at least 50% of seropositive recipients who receive an allograft from a seropositive donor [6] – the incidence of symptomatic HCMV infection in seropositive recipients of allografts from seropositive donors is 30–50%, depending on the organ being transplanted [6]

Table 1.2. *TNF, tumour necrosis factor.*

the cardiovascular system, including impaired vascular function [9] and increased risk of atherosclerosis. It has also been associated with restenosis following balloon angioplasty [10,11].

The replication of HCMV is very effectively controlled in the immunocompetent host and the absence of an effective T-cell immune response is central to the pathogenesis of HCMV disease [3]. Consequently, HCMV is an important cause of morbidity and mortality in individuals whose immune system is immature (eg, neonates) or suppressed because of therapeutic drugs or disease. The latter category includes:

- patients with human immunodeficiency virus (HIV)/acquired immune deficiency syndrome (AIDS), leukaemia or lymphoma;
- cancer patients undergoing chemotherapy;
- patients who have undergone solid organ or stem cell transplantation; and
- other patients receiving immunosuppressive therapy.

Three phases of the HCMV replication cycle
Immediate-early (IE) phase
• Transcription of the IE or alpha (α) genes occurs in the first 4 hours following viral infection • Nonstructural proteins appear in the nucleus within 4 hours after infection [5] • This phase results in the synthesis of proteins that regulate the expression of the remaining viral genes and also manipulate cellular processes
Early (E) phase
• Transcription of the E or beta (β) genes • A variety of essential viral proteins are produced: most notably, viral enzymes and proteins involved in viral DNA replication, including the DNA polymerase and helicase-primase
Late (L) phase
• L or gamma (γ) gene products are made within approximately 24 hours after infection • Virally encoded structural proteins appear in the nucleus and cytoplasm within 6–24 hours after DNA synthesis [5] • Synthesis of L gene products is highly dependent on viral DNA replication and can be blocked by inhibitors of viral DNA polymerase, such as ganciclovir • Once structural proteins have been produced, the entire virion is assembled and new infectious virus is released

Table 2.1.

Defining HCMV dynamics in the human host

On the basis of the groundbreaking work performed in the mid-1990s to define HIV-1 replication *in vivo*, similar approaches have been adopted to define the replication dynamics of HCMV *in vivo*. Using a series of AIDS patients who had experienced long periods of HCMV replication prior to the diagnosis of retinitis and whose HCMV viral load patterns indicated that the replication HCMV was in a steady state, frequent serial HCMV load measures following treatment were used to accurately measure the decline rate. The results showed that the half-life (and therefore doubling time at steady state) was approximately 1 day [18]. The half-life of viral load decline after initiation of antiviral therapy has been shown to affect treatment response in transplant recipients with HCMV infection (*see* Table 2.2) [20]. In addition, other risk factors for the response of HCMV to therapy included viral load at the initiation of therapy and virus doubling time before therapy. Using similar approaches, it has been shown that the half-life of decline following therapy with intravenous ganciclovir (5 mg/kg bid) or valganciclovir (900 mg bid) is essentially the same (*see* Figure 2.3).

HCMV load and mortality

The risk of developing HCMV disease and death in individuals with advanced AIDS has been reported to be directly related to the quantity of HCMV DNA in plasma and whole blood, and in these patients, HCMV load is a better predictor of outcome than CD4 lymphocyte count [21]. In addition, a prospective study to investigate whether HCMV viraemia remains a significant risk factor for progression of HIV disease and death in the era of highly active antiretroviral therapy (HAART) showed that detection of HCMV in blood by PCR continues to identify HIV-infected patients with a poor prognosis [22]. Randomised controlled clin-

Univariable risk factors for HCMV response to therapy

Risk factors	Odds ratio	CI 95% for odds ratio	*p* value
Initial viral load (per $\log_{10}$ higher)	2.39	1.05–5.44	0.038
Doubling time of viral load (per day increase)	2.95	1.28–6.82	0.01
Half-life of viral decline (per day increase)	3.01	1.45–6.25	0.003

Table 2.2. *CI, confidence interval. Data taken from Mattes* et al *[20].*

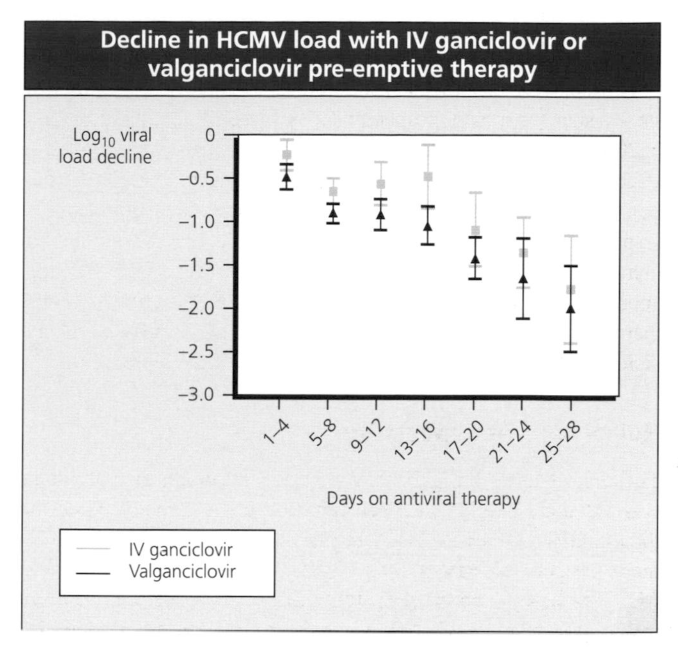

Figure 2.3.

ical trials of drugs active against HCMV are needed to investigate whether asymptomatic viraemia is a marker or a determinant of HIV disease progression [22]. In a further prospective study involving patients with AIDS seropositive for HCMV, detection of HCMV viraemia was predictive of death and provided additional prognostic information on the risk of all-cause mortality beyond that obtained with CD4 cell count and HIV viral load testing alone [23]. An ancillary study of a randomised, placebo-controlled, phase III clinical trial was conducted to determine the association of HCMV viraemia with mortality and HCMV retinitis progression in newly diagnosed and relapsed HCMV retinitis [24]. This study showed that in patients with AIDS and HCMV retinitis, the detection of plasma HCMV DNA was associated with a higher risk of mortality compared with a high HIV viral load. Anti-HCMV therapy provided a transient reduction in HCMV viraemia in newly diagnosed, but not relapsed, patients with HCMV retinitis [24].

A case–cohort study showed that HCMV viraemia in the first year after paediatric primary lung transplantation is associated with increased risk of death or re-transplantation between 90 and 365 days post-transplant when HCMV prophylaxis has stopped [25].

Host immune response against HCMV

The human host mounts a vigorous immune response against HCMV. A number of antigens are targets of the adaptive immune response, which involves both antibody and T-cell-mediated immune responses. In addition, innate immune responses also play an important role in protection [26].

B-cell immune responses

Although a number of proteins from HCMV elicit an antibody response (ie, envelope glycoproteins, proteins from the tegument, capsid, and nonstructural proteins), it appears that only a small number of surface glycoproteins are important in generating a neutralising antibody response. The best characterised protein is glycoprotein B (gB), which is involved in the early stages of viral attachment through its binding to heparin sulphate molecules on the cell surface; it can further bind Toll-like receptor-2 [27]. It has been estimated that up to 50% of the host neutralising antibody response is accounted for by responses to gB, with the majority of the neutralising antibodies recognising a small (about 70 amino acids) but complex region of the protein termed AD-1. In addition, neutralising antibodies against gH and the glycoprotein M/N complex have also been documented (for a comprehensive review on the glycoproteins of HCMV, *see* Britt *et al* [28]). A monoclonal antibody targeted at a single neutralising site in gH has been used for therapy in AIDS patients and stem cell transplant patients with HCMV infection, but with limited clinical success [29,30]. The clinical significance of neutralising antibodies against gB has not been fully elucidated in the human host, but neutralising antibodies in animal models can limit virus spread (even in the absence of effective T-cells) [31]. In the guinea pig system, immunisation with gB substantially reduces foetal disease following inoculation of a pregnant animal with a fully virulent strain of guinea pig cytomegalovirus [32,33].

T-cell immune responses

The human host devotes a substantial proportion of its T-cell immune system to the control of HCMV replication. Recent data using overlapping peptides have revealed that the majority of the HCMV proteome is targeted by the T-cell arm of the immune system, although certain key proteins elicit dominant responses in the majority of human subjects tested to date [34]. These proteins include pp65 (the same protein detected by the antigenaemia assay) and the immediate-early protein IE-1, together with gB. Using class I HLA tetramer reagents it has been shown that CD8 T-cell frequencies against a single epitope in pp65 can reach 1–5% in healthy immunocompetent individuals, and this proportion can increase in patients with active, high-level replication to about 40% in some cases [35,36]. These CD8 T-cells appear to have the characteristics of terminally differentiated CD8 cells in that they are fully able to kill targets and are granzyme and perforin positive [37]. Interestingly, there is little evidence for extensive immune escape occurring through mutations within these epitopes. CD8 T-cell memory against HCMV is maintained in cells bearing both the CD45RO and CD45RA phenotype, which is unusual [38]. There is increasing evidence for a substantial expansion of the HCMV CD8 T-cell response as the human host gets older [39]. The implications of this observation for the control of other infections and neoplasias has not been fully elucidated, but it has been noted that very old individuals with a large expansion of HCMV CD8 T-cells have a shorter survival time compared with age-matched controls not exhibiting this phenotype [40,41].

CD4 responses against HCMV are equally substantial and appear to be important for the control of HCMV replication mediated through effector CD8 T-cells [42,43]. Thus, in HIV-infected patients, significant reductions in CD4 T-cells against HCMV are associated with increased viral replication, despite the presence of CD8 T-cells. At later stages of HIV infection, the ability of these HCMV CD8 T-cells to secrete IFN-γ following peptide stimulation appears to be compromised and correlates with the appearance of clinically overt retinitis [44]. HAART has been shown to lead to the immune reconstitution of CD4 T-cells against HCMV and, consequently, allow control of replication through normal CD8 T-cell effector functions, although whether these responses return to normal is debatable [45].

Immune manipulation by HCMV

Given the substantial immune response generated against HCMV, it is perhaps not surprising that the virus has evolved a number of mechanisms to manipulate and evade the immune response [46–48]. These include a variety of ways to downregulate class I HLA display, the possession of a number of chemokine and cytokine homologues, various class I HLA structural mimics involved in natural killer cell subversion, as well as chemokine receptors. These proteins are summarised in Table 3.1.

The variety of gene products used by HCMV to manipulate the host immune response to HCMV infection

Function	HCMV gene
Class I HLA display/presentation	
Cause proteasomal degradation of immediate-early-1 protein	pp65 (*UL83*)
Interrupt the function of the transporter associated with peptide translocation	*US6*
Retain class I HLA heavy chains in the ER	*US3*
Redirect class I HLA heavy chains for degradation	*US2/US11*
Interfere with class II HLA	*US2/US3*
Class I HLA heavy chain homologues	*UL18/UL141/UL142*
NK cell manipulation	
Enhance presentation of HLA-E to NKG2D receptors in infected cells	*UL40*
Antagonise NK receptor CD226/96	*UL141/UL16*
Viral chemokines/cytokines	
Viral IL-10 homologue	*UL111.5A*
Viral CXC chemokine	*UL146/Ul147*
Viral chemokine/cytokine receptors	
Chemokine receptor homologues	*US27/US28/UL33/UL78*
TNF receptor homologue	*UL144*

Table 3.1. *HLA, human leukocyte antigen; ER, endoplasmic reticulum; NK, natural killer; TNF, tumour necrosis factor.*

Diagnosis of HCMV infection

The majority of primary infections with HCMV remain undiagnosed because the virus usually produces few, if any, symptoms in immunocompetent hosts. However, rapid and accurate methods for diagnosing HCMV infection are essential because of the substantial health impact of HCMV disease on neonates and immunocompromised individuals. Laboratory tests to detect the presence of IgG antibodies to HCMV – these persist in the body for the lifetime of the infected individual – can be used to determine prior infection, and measuring the avidity index of the IgG antibodies can be used as a marker of recent infection (IgG antibodies have low avidity during the early phases of infection and then mature to high avidity as the primary infection progresses). In addition, primary infection can also be identified through the presence of antibodies of the IgM class. It is worth noting that while serology is excellent for determining the serostatus of patients prior to organ transplantation, IgG measurements have virtually no role to play following transplantation due to the influence of immunosuppressive therapy. Hence, direct detection of HCMV – via assays such as the PCR or antigenaemia – is necessary for optimal patient management and to monitor the effects of antiviral therapy [6].

Historically, diagnosis of HCMV disease has been made by histopathology, where cytomegalic inclusions can be recognised in biopsy material by the typical 'owl-eyes' appearance (*see* Figure 4.1); however, this approach necessitates an invasive procedure to obtain samples [4]. Furthermore, the diagnosis of invasive disease is complicated because the level of HCMV replication in the target organ needed to produce 'owl-eyes' inclusion is high, whereas lower levels that do not yield inclusions may still be pathologically important. Immunohistochemistry is often a useful adjunct in the diagnosis of tissue-invasive HCMV infection. The diagnosis of HCMV-associated disease should be based on relevant clinical signs and symptoms of disease and detection of virus in blood or from the involved tissue (with the exception of retinitis) [3].

HCMV infection following renal transplantation

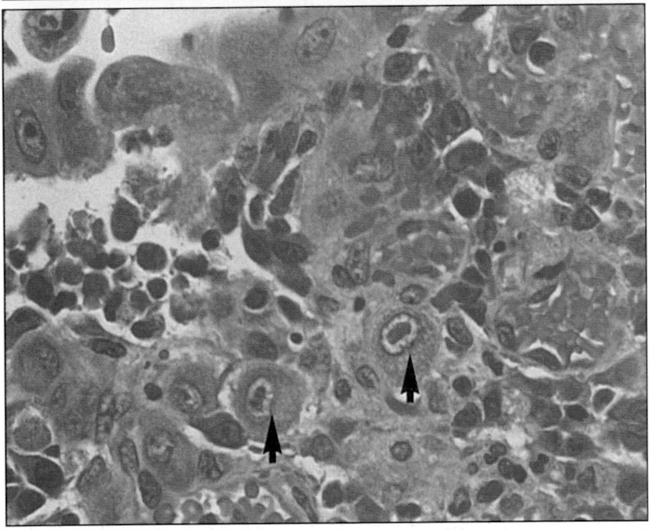

Figure 4.1. *HCMV inclusions surrounded by a clear halo and thickened nuclear membrane (arrows), rendering an 'owl's eye' appearance to the infected cell.*

Diagnostic assays for the direct detection of HCMV replication

The role of virological assays

Several assays have been developed for diagnosis and monitoring of HCMV infection in immunocompromised patients [3]. The most widely used assays measure viraemia, antigenaemia, DNA and mRNA [3,5,6,49]. The goal of virological assays is to enable earlier diagnosis of infection and more rapid provision of results to physicians to permit optimal patient management.

Viral cultures (viraemia)

- For many years, culture-based methods have been considered the gold standard for diagnosis of HCMV infection:

  - the endpoint is a characteristic cytopathic effect produced by productive replication of HCMV in human fibroblast cultures and routinely takes 2–4 weeks.
- HCMV can be cultured from a variety of body fluids including urine, tissues, bronchoalveolar lavage fluid, saliva and blood.
- The first rapid culture-based assays comprised inoculation of human fibroblasts with the clinical sample followed by a 16- to 24-hour incubation and then immunohistochemical detection of HCMV proteins (the shell vial assay or the detection of early antigen fluorescent foci assay).
- Viraemia (detection of HCMV in peripheral blood leukocytes and whole blood) has better prognostic value for disease than detection of virus in other fluids, such as urine and saliva.
- Conventional culture assays lack sensitivity for detecting active replication in blood, and are not optimal for guiding pre-emptive therapy for HCMV infection since they do not allow quantification of viral load and have a limited degree of reproducibility [15].
- Cell culture-based assays are being superseded by PCR and antigenaemia assays, but may be useful in isolating HCMV strains for resistance testing.

Antigenaemia

- Assay uses monoclonal antibodies to detect pp65, a 65-kDa structural phosphoprotein present in peripheral blood leukocytes during active HCMV infection [50].
- Provides an early, indirect marker of active HCMV infection and is a rapid test for detection of HCMV viraemia:
  - the magnitude of viral load can be estimated from the number of pp65-positive leukocytes [50].
- Highly sensitive and specific for the diagnosis of HCMV infection:
  - prognostic value of the assay is superior to cell culture-based methods.

- Reliable, rapid.
- Quantitative antigenaemia can be used to predict HCMV disease and to monitor response to antiviral therapy.
- Disadvantages with antigenaemia (compared with PCR) are:
  - interpretation is subjective and may impact on standardisation and precision (flow cytometry has been applied to automate the technique and thereby make it less subjective) [51];
  - blood collected for these assays must be processed within 6–8 hours [4]; and
  - unsuitable for processing very large numbers of blood samples for HCMV detection.

Measurement of DNA (DNAemia)

- For the qualitative and quantitative detection of viral DNA in blood.
- Uses PCR or other hybridisation techniques.
- Qualitative PCR on whole blood, isolated peripheral blood leukocytes and plasma is a rapid, sensitive and easily automated technique.
- Quantitative DNAemia has been shown to correlate with virus replication and clinical symptoms.
- Quantitative PCR is used in the clinical setting to identify patients at risk of developing HCMV disease, to provide rapid diagnosis of established HCMV disease and to predict the risk of virological and clinical relapse [15].
- Quantitative PCR can also be used to monitor response to antiviral therapy and is useful as a surrogate marker of clinical or viral resistance.
- Although all components within blood provide excellent prognostic information, whole blood, rather than plasma or other blood compartments, may provide the optimal sample for HCMV DNA quantification [52–55].
- HCMV DNA detection in dried blood spots on Guthrie cards may be a powerful tool for diagnosing congenital infection retrospectively [56]:

  - dried blood spots can be pooled and tested in batches without losing sensitivity, thereby reducing screening costs [57]; and
  - stored samples may be used to diagnose congenital HCMV infection [58].

Measurement of viral mRNA (RNAemia)

- To detect a virus product more directly related to virus replication than DNA.
- The technique used is nucleic acid sequence-based amplification – an isothermal reaction that permits amplification of unspliced viral mRNA in a background of DNA.
- The pp67 mRNA transcript is routinely used for detection.
- Samples of whole blood, isolated peripheral blood leukocytes or buffy coat can be used and can provide prognostic information.

For more than a decade, routine use of quantitative PCR along with antigenaemia and viraemia has enabled optimal control and monitoring of HCMV infections and antiviral treatment in immunocompromised individuals [49]. Evidence of viraemia using antigenaemia or PCR is often found several days and sometimes weeks before the onset of clinical symptoms, thereby providing the opportunity to initiate therapy in the absence of the direct effects of HCMV. Although the virological assays described above were developed for the diagnosis and monitoring of HCMV infection in immunocompromised patients, they have also been useful for the study of HCMV kinetics in immunocompetent individuals during the convalescent phase of a primary infection [59].

The role of serological assays pretransplant

Serological assays (in both the donor and recipient) are useful for identifying HCMV risk at the time of transplant and documenting seroconversion of a previously seronegative patient [4]. The value of serology is limited to pre-transplantation, however, as serological techniques are not as useful in diagnosing clinical disease or for monitoring antiviral therapy as the virological assays, which enable earlier, more accurate diagnosis and more rapid results.

Measurement of antibody to HCMV

- Highly specific and sensitive in immunocompetent individuals.
- Presence of anti-HCMV antibodies indicates previous infection, but does not specify the level of immunity.
- Enzyme-linked immunosorbent assay (ELISA) is the most commonly available serological test for measuring antibody to HCMV [51].
- Other methods for detecting HCMV IgG include latex agglutination, radioimmunoassay, complement-fixation test and immunofluorescence tests.
- Serological assays are not recommended for monitoring HCMV infection in immunocompromised individuals, as results can be unreliable.
- Diagnosis of primary infection in pregnancy has improved greatly with the introduction of IgG avidity assays [60].

Recommendations for diagnosis of HCMV infection in transplant recipients

The latest International Herpes Management Forum (IHMF®; www.ihmf.org) recommendations for the diagnosis and monitoring of HCMV infection in solid organ and haematopoietic stem cell transplant recipients are shown in Table 4.1 [15].

IHMF® recommendations for diagnosis and monitoring of HCMV infection in transplant recipients
• HCMV load measurements can be used to monitor response to therapy and to predict the time required to reduce CMV load to undetectable levels (category 1 statement)
• Although detection of HCMV by PCR in many compartments of blood (eg, plasma, leukocytes) can provide prognostic information, HCMV DNA levels in whole blood are significantly higher than those present in plasma, so whole blood should be the sample of choice (category 1 recommendation)

Table 4.1. *Continued overleaf.*

IHMF® recommendations for diagnosis and monitoring of HCMV infection in transplant recipients
• Owing to the rapid dynamics of HCMV, a randomised, controlled trial is needed to determine the optimum sampling frequency for quantitative measures of viral load (research need recommendation) • An international quantitation standard distributed by an external quality-control organisation is required to compare studies using different PCR-based systems and to facilitate patient management at multiple care centres (research need recommendation)
Recommendations and statement categories
The IHMF® publishes management recommendations and statements under four categories, which are: *Category 1* Consistent evidence from controlled clinical trials. For example, for an antiviral this would include results from at least one well-designed, randomised, controlled clinical trial, and, in the case of laboratory studies, consistent evidence from comparative studies *Category 2* Evidence from at least one well-designed clinical trial without randomisation, from cohort or case-controlled analytical studies (preferably from more than one centre), or from multiple time-series studies or dramatic results from uncontrolled experiments *Category 3* Evidence from opinions of respected authorities based on clinical experience, descriptive studies or reports of expert committees *Research need* Area in which research is warranted

Table 4.1. *(Continued). Reproduced with permission from Razonable and Emery [15].*

Direct effects of HCMV infection

Cellular effects

HCMV can infect a wide variety of cells in the body, including dendritic cells, endothelial cells, epithelial cells, hepatocytes, peripheral blood leukocytes and smooth muscle cells [61–64]. Specialised parenchymal cells, such as neurones in the brain and retina, can also be infected with the virus. Cells infected with HCMV often become enlarged (cytomegalia) and show intranuclear inclusions. Latent infection is maintained primarily in secretory glands, lymphoreticular cells and the kidneys, with bone marrow progenitor cells being a major site of latency [65]. HCMV has evolved a number of genes that allow the virus to manipulate a range of cellular processes involved in cell-cycle control and apoptosis, presumably to create a cellular environment that allows the virus to complete its replication cycle in an efficient and timely fashion [66].

Immunocompetent individuals

In immunocompetent children, adolescents and adults, most primary HCMV infections are predominantly associated with mild clinical symptoms such as headache, fatigue and sore throat, and rarely cause serious illness [67,68]. Some healthy individuals infected with HCMV may experience mild symptoms similar to those of infectious mononucleosis, including prolonged fever, fatigue, myalgia, pharyngitis, mild hepatitis, splenic enlargement and lymphadenopathy [5]. This mononucleosis-like syndrome, which is often called the 'HCMV syndrome', is indistinguishable from primary Epstein–Barr virus infection [3]. Symptoms resembling a mild, glandular fever-like illness are essentially clinically insignificant unless they occur during pregnancy. Less common complications of primary HCMV infection include arthralgia and arthritis, ulcerative colitis, pneumonitis, Guillain–Barré syndrome, aseptic meningitis and myocarditis [3]. However, it should be noted that children with subclinical infection, who are potentially excreting large quantities of virus for extended periods of time, are a primary source of HCMV transmission to their parents. This is clinically significant if the mother is pregnant and also seronegative for HCMV.

In contrast to primary infection, active infection caused by reactivation of latent virus appears to be asymptomatic [49]. The role played by re-infections (ie, infections by a new virus strain in an immunocompetent individual) remains to be determined [49].

Neonates

Congenital HCMV infection and disease

HCMV is the virus most commonly transmitted to the developing child *in utero* and is an important cause of congenital viral infection. In the USA, for example, HCMV infection affects from 0.2% to more than 3% of all live births (*see* Table 5.1). Congenital HCMV disease is clinically important and can lead to death of a foetus or a premature birth. Congenital HCMV infection can follow both pri-

Estimated annual public health impact of congenital HCMV in the USA and UK

	USA	UK
Number of live births	4,000,000	700,000
Proportion congenitally infected	1%	0.3%
Number of congenitally infected	40,000	2100
Number of cytomegalic inclusion disease (7%)	2800	147
Number of fatal (12%)	336	18
Number of with sequelae (90%)	2218	132
Number of asymptomatic (93%)	37,200	1953
Number of with sequelae (15%)	5580	293
Total number damaged	8134	443

Table 5.1. *Reproduced with permission from Griffiths [69].*

mary and recurrent maternal infections, although it is mainly related to primary maternal infection [8,70]. In a population-based study, maternal immunity to HCMV prior to conception has been shown to provide substantial protection (69%) against congenital viral infection [71]. The risk after birth of HCMV-related complications in infected infants appears to be mostly associated with women who have not been previously infected with HCMV (seronegative) and become infected for the first time during pregnancy (0.7–4% of women) [72]. Primary HCMV infection of seronegative mothers during pregnancy is associated with a 30–40% risk of intrauterine transmission, and adverse outcome is more likely when infection occurs within the first half of gestation [73].

Approximately, 7% of infected neonates at birth have symptoms of cytomegalic inclusion disease, including microcephaly, encephalitis, hepatosplenomegaly, thrombocytopenic purpura, hearing loss and intracranial calcifications [74]. Neonates with such symptoms have a very poor prognosis. In addition, a further 15% of asymptomatic HCMV-infected neonates will subsequently develop disease [74]. Common HCMV-related complications in infected infants include hearing loss, visual impairment, and diminished mental and motor capabilities. The risk of developing hearing loss or mental retardation continues for many years [75]. Up to 80% of congenitally infected infants born with symptoms are estimated to exhibit serious life-long neurological abnormalities, with severe life-threatening organ dysfunction and death occurring in 10–20% of patients [3]. Sensorineural hearing loss (SNHL) in congenital HCMV affects 40–60% of symptomatic infants and 7–15% of asymptomatic infants [76,77]. SNHL ranges from mild unilateral to profound bilateral hearing loss, and may be progressive or fluctuating. The onset of HCMV-induced hearing loss may not occur until after the neonatal period, but it usually falls within the critical period for speech and language development [74,78,79].

One of the first demonstrations that viral load was an important marker for pathogenesis was provided in 1975 by Alford and Stagno, who showed, using conventional cell culture approaches, that the viral load in the urine of congenitally infected neonates was highest in those with symptoms [12]. With the advent of more sensitive methods for detection and quantification, such as PCR, many centres will measure viral load in a congenitally infected infant to gauge the likely risk of symptomatology. A further extension of this approach has been to determine HCMV load in amniotic fluid during the early period of pregnancy (weeks 18–20). Lazzarotto and colleagues have clearly demonstrated that transmission is related to the viral load in the amniotic fluid, and higher levels of HCMV replication evidenced by high HCMV loads increases the risk for congenital disease at birth [80,81].

Perinatal HCMV infection and disease

The clinical presentation of HCMV disease in neonates who are infected perinatally differs depending on the gestational period of the infant. In premature neonates deprived of passively acquired maternal-specific immunoglobulin G (IgG) antibodies, perinatal HCMV infection can mimic sepsis, whereas in full-term neonates it is usually clinically benign [74,82,83]. Perinatal HCMV infection should not be ignored in full-term infants, however, because this could lead to misdiagnosis of congenital HCMV in a child being investigated for hearing loss or mental retardation [74].

Immunocompromised individuals

Since the integrity of the T-cell arm of the immune system is paramount in the control of HCMV replication, the T-cell immunocompromised individual experiencing both primary and reactivated HCMV infections is likely to suffer more severe clinical consequences compared with immunocompetent subjects [67,84]. Primary HCMV infection or reactivation of latent virus can cause serious disease in different organ systems – most often in the eyes, lungs or liver – and may lead to death. Retinitis (which may result in blindness), pneumonia and gastrointestinal disease are common manifestations of HCMV disease and are often accompanied by fever and mononucleosis-like symptoms. Polyradiculopathy and encephalopathy are also observed, especially in HIV-infected patients prior to the widespread use of HAART. The range of clinical manifestations associated with HCMV in the immunocompromised host is summarised in Table 5.2. Prolonged fever is a common manifestation in solid organ transplant patients, whereas pneumonitis and

Relative occurrence of different HCMV diseases in the immunocompromised host

Symptoms	Solid organ transplant	Bone marrow transplant	AIDS
Fever/hepatitis	++	+	+
Gastrointestinal	+	+	+
Retinitis	+	+	++
Pneumonitis	+	++	N/A
Myelosuppression	N/A	++	N/A
Encephalopathy	N/A	N/A	+
Polyradiculopathy	N/A	N/A	+
Addisonian state	N/A	N/A	+
Immunosuppression	+	N/A	N/A
Rejection	+	N/A	N/A

Table 5.2. *+, diseases that occur in the designated patient population; ++, diseases that are most common. AIDS, acquired immunodeficiency syndrome; N/A, not associated.*

retinitis are the most frequently observed in stem cell transplant and AIDS patients, respectively.

The international definitions for HCMV end-organ disease are shown in Table 5.3. In the absence of antiviral prophylaxis, HCMV infection occurs primarily within the first 3 months following solid organ transplantation. However, in patients receiving prophylaxis for 3 months, the majority of infections that occur will be delayed to the period following prophylaxis [4,86]. Prior to the widespread use of prophylaxis for HCMV and the use of efficient laboratory methods to monitor patients for replication, the risk of symptomatic disease in D^+R^- solid organ transplant recipient could easily reach 60% or higher. HCMV disease rates tend to be highest in heart–lung recipients (39–41%) and lowest in kidney transplant recipients (8–32%) [87,88]. The consequences of HCMV disease are similar in all solid organ transplant patients, although specific organ involvement by HCMV often corresponds to the organ transplanted [50]. Fever has

International definitions for HCMV end organ disease

Disease	Definition
Pneumonia (transplant recipients)	Radiographic changes and/or hypoxia HCMV detected in BAL or lung biopsy
Pneumonia (HIV-infected individuals)	Symptoms of pneumonia with hypoxaemia HCMV detected in the lung Absence of other pathogens
Gastrointestinal	Gastrointestinal symptoms with HCMV detected by histology
Hepatitis	Abnormal liver function tests, histological changes and HCMV detection in liver biopsy
Neurological	Symptoms of encephalitis, transverse myelitis, or other CNS symptoms, plus HCMV in CSF
Retinitis	Typical ophthalmological lesions without virological proof

Table 5.3. *BAL, bronchoalveolar lavage; CNS, central nervous system; CSF, cerebrospinal fluid; HCMV, human cytomegalovirus; HIV, human immunodeficiency virus. Adapted from Llungman* et al *[85].*

been associated with more severe forms of HCMV disease in a study of kidney transplant recipients, and was suggested by the study authors to be important in assessing the severity and prognosis of the HCMV disease [89].

HCMV-associated pneumonitis is characterised by increasing hypoxia and progression to respiratory failure [3]. Pneumonitis following allogeneic stem cell transplantation is associated with a mortality of 60–80% without ganciclovir antiviral therapy, and 50% when treated with antiviral therapy plus HCMV hyperimmunoglobulin [26,51].

HCMV is one of the most important opportunistic pathogens in patients infected with HIV. Clinical disease due to HCMV has been recognised in up to 40% of patients with advanced HIV disease [51]. More than 90% of cases of HCMV among patients with AIDS are due to reactivation of endogenous virus. Declining CD4 T-cell function against HCMV due to the HIV-1-mediated destruction of

HCMV-specific CD4 T-cells and the consequent derangement of the CD8 response allows HCMV replication to reach high levels and remain at these levels for some considerable time before the expression of HCMV disease occurs. Before the introduction of HAART, HCMV disease in AIDS patients was associated with a range of adverse conditions, including retinitis (observed in up to 40% of patients and characterised by haemorrhagic retinal necrosis), gastrointestinal disease, polyradiculopathy, encephalitis and adrenalitis. The diagnosis of HCMV disease was associated with a particularly poor prognosis [49,90]. The advent of HAART has reduced the risk of HCMV disease, improved prognosis for patients infected with HIV and decreased mortality from AIDS, in addition to changing the clinical picture of HIV-associated eye disease [91]. As well as reducing HIV load, HAART is also effective in achieving immune reconstitution, thus tipping the balance back in favour of the host immune system to control HCMV replication [45,92]. In HIV-infected patients with active HCMV replication, the immune reconstitution following HAART is usually sufficient to bring HCMV replication under control without the requirement of anti-HCMV therapy [93].

6

Indirect effects of HCMV infection

In addition to the significant morbidity directly attributable to HCMV as an infectious pathogen, the virus has also been associated with several clinical conditions, collectively termed 'indirect effects' [84]. It is unclear whether high viral loads are associated with the indirect effects of HCMV and it is conceivable that periods of asymptomatic viraemia may also predispose the host to the longer term manifestations grouped within the indirect effects category. The indirect effects may be mediated in a large part by the production of cytokines, chemokines and growth factors by the host in response to viral replication and tissue invasion. However, the HCMV genome itself encodes a number of homologues of chemokines together with cytokines and chemokine receptors, which may also contribute to the expression of these indirect effects [6,94,95]. An overview comparing the mechanisms of the direct and indirect effects of HCMV is shown in Figure 6.1.

Solid organ transplantation

It has been postulated that many of the complications of HCMV infection in solid organ transplantation are caused by indirect effects of the virus, including acute and chronic graft rejection, graft-versus-host disease, superinfection by other viruses, bacteria and fungi, opportunistic neoplasms, accelerated atherosclerosis after heart transplant and death (*see* Table 6.1) [6,97–99]. Clearly, each of these conditions is multifactorial, but there is evidence to indicate that HCMV makes an active contribution to their pathogenesis [98].

The consequences of the immunomodulatory effects of HCMV are considerable. In patients undergoing solid organ transplantation, active HCMV infection has been shown to be an independent risk factor for the development of other infectious complications, including bacteraemia and invasive fungal disease [101–103]. HCMV infection is correlated with an increased incidence of:

- septicaemia with *Listeria monocytogenes*, *Candida* spp. and a variety of Gram-negative bacilli;

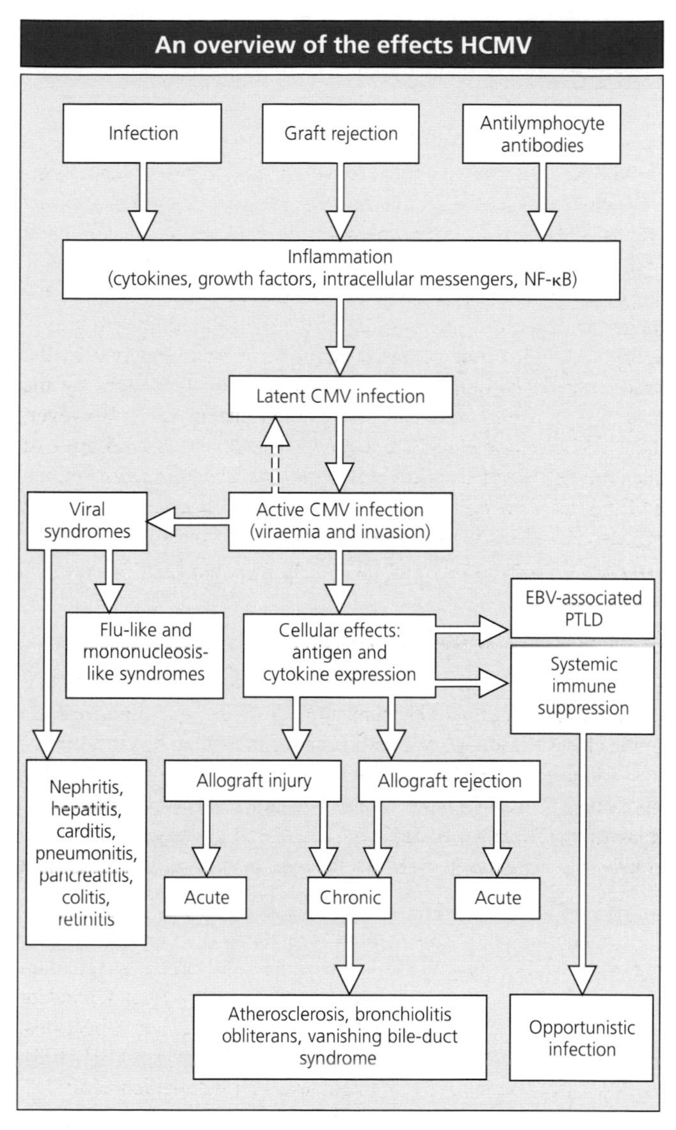

Figure 6.1. *EBV, Epstein–Barr virus; PTLD, post-traumatic lymphoproliferative disease. Reproduced with permission from Fishman* et al *[96].*

Indirect effects of HCMV in solid organ transplant recipients
• An immunomodulating effect, such that the net state of immunosuppression is beyond that induced by immunosuppressive drugs: – this effect may predispose the patient to infection with opportunistic microorganisms, including other viruses, bacteria and fungi – post-transplant lymphoproliferative disease may be elevated in patients with HCMV infections
• Acute and/or chronic allograft injury
• Potential increased risk of acute and chronic rejection of allografts: – HCMV has been associated with the development of acute and chronic rejection via mechanisms of enhanced allorecognition
• Allograft dysfunction and decreased survival

Table 6.1. *Adapted from Rubin [84] and Paya [100].*

- *Pneumocyctis jiroveci (carinii)* pneumonia, invasive pulmonary aspergillosis and colonisation of the upper respiratory tract with Gram-negative bacilli;
- reactivation of toxoplasmosis; and
- a significant increase in the viral load of a range of viruses, such as hepatitis C virus, HHV-6 and HIV.

HCMV may also interact with other viruses, resulting in accelerated hepatitis C virus pathogenesis and increased incidence of Epstein–Barr virus-associated post-transplant lymphoproliferative disease.

HCMV infection has been implicated in the development of acute and chronic allograft injury, both of which are associated with decreased allograft function and patient survival [4,84,104–106]. The relationship between HCMV and allograft injury is bidirectional [107,108]. Cytokines, chemokines and growth factors are induced in response to both HCMV infection and allograft rejection, resulting in activation of the vascular endothelium and inflammatory cells [108]. The proinflammatory cytokine TNF-α is a key mediator in reactivating HCMV from latency (*see* Table 1.2). TNF-α-induced activation of protein kinase C and nuclear factor-κB (NF-κB) lead to the expression of HCMV immediate-early proteins, which trigger the onset of viral replication (*see* Table 2.1). As TNF-α is released during allograft rejection, HCMV reactivation in response to acute rejection is also likely to contribute to the complexity of distinguishing whether HCMV infection is causing the allograft rejection, is a consequence of the rejection episode, or is contributing to and perhaps exacerbating the rejection [108]. In this context, intensive augmented immunosuppressive therapy to treat rejection episodes can facilitate viral replication, turning an asymptomatic viraemic episode into a symptomatic one; for example, the incidence of HCMV disease may increase up to fivefold following treatment with antilymphocyte agents [96].

Several mechanisms have been proposed for HCMV-related allograft rejection [5]. For example, HCMV infection of the vascular endothelium and smooth muscle cells has been suggested to play an important role in the pathogenesis of vascular injury observed in acute and chronic rejection [108]. Other mechanisms that may influence allograft rejection include: regulation of major histocompatibility complex (MHC) II molecules in the allograft [109,110]; upregulation of adhesion molecules on allograft endothelium and their ligands on leukocytes; and release of cytokines [108,111–113]. HCMV upregulates endothelial adhesion molecules, such as vascular cell adhesion molecule (VCAM-1), intercellular adhesion molecule (ICAM-1), lymphocyte function-associated antigen 1 (LFA-1) and very late antigen 4 (VLA-4), which may increase the number of inflammatory cells in the graft [108]. Furthermore, endothelitis and endothelial proliferation caused by direct cytopathic effects or by the action of anti-endothelial cell antibodies (induced by HCMV [108]) has been shown to trigger allograft rejection [5,114]. HCMV infection is an independent risk factor for acute kidney graft rejection and is also associated with increased long-term mortality and post-transplant diabetes mellitus in renal transplant recipients [17]. In a comprehensive study of 160 consecutive non-diabetic renal transplant recipients by Hjelmesaeth and colleagues [115], asymptomatic HCMV infection was associated with a significant increase in the incidence of new-onset diabetes (26.2% vs 6.3% in patients with no evidence of HCMV replication). In a multivariable analysis, both asymptomatic infection (odds ratio, 4.00; p=0.025) and age (odds ratio, 1.04; p=0.05) were the only factors associated with new-onset, post-transplant diabetes. Interestingly, first-phase insulin secretion was significantly lower in patients with asymptomatic HCMV infection, as were second-phase secretion and area under the concentration (AUC) for insulin secretion.

HCMV remains one of the most important pathogens following lung transplantation, with the indirect effects of the virus leading to long-term adverse sequelae in the lung allograft [108]. There is increasing evidence to indicate that the indirect effects of HCMV may be at least as important as its direct effects in terms of morbidity and mortality in this transplant population [108].

HCMV may also contribute to chronic graft vasculopathy, resulting in lesions such as chronic allograft nephropathy (in kidney transplant recipients), bronchiolitis obliterans (in lung transplant recipients; a major limiting factor to long-term survival after lung transplantation [108]), vanishing bile duct syndrome (in liver transplant recipients), and accelerated coronary artery disease (in heart transplant recipients) [4,15,88,116]. HCMV infection and disease have been shown to increase the length of hospital stay and the overall cost of care of solid organ transplant recipients [50,108].

HCMV may be a potential pathogen in atherosclerosis and its clinical manifestations through either direct effects on vascular wall cells (eg, cell lysis and proinflammatory changes) or indirect systemic effects, which may involve induction of acute-phase proteins, establishment of a prothrombotic state, haemodynamic stress caused by tachycardia, increased cardiac output or a regional inflammatory activation in response to systemic endotoxaemia and cytokinaemia [117].

Haematopoietic stem cell transplantation

Indirect immunomodulatory effects of HCMV are being increasingly recognised in haematopoietic stem cell transplant recipients [118–120]. For example, a study to assess the impact of donor and recipient HCMV serostatus on mortality after allogeneic non-T-cell-depleted stem cell transplantation showed that HCMV serostatus remains an important factor associated with mortality, and HCMV disease was associated with mortality among seropositive recipients. However, in seronegative recipients of transplants from seropositive donors, mortality was attributable to bacterial and fungal infection, which was consistent with the immunomodulatory effects of HCMV infection [121]. HCMV-induced CD13-specific autoimmunity has been suggested to contribute to tissue damage in chronic graft-versus-host reactions [122]. An association between HCMV infection and the development of Guillain–Barré syndrome in the setting of allogeneic haematopoietic stem cell transplantation has also been reported [123]. Increased levels of TNF-α have also been associated with an increased risk of HCMV infection after allogeneic haematopoietic stem cell transplantation [124].

AIDS

In patients infected with HIV, HCMV can exert indirect effects that accelerate progression to AIDS and death [3]. A high HCMV viral load in AIDS patients is associated with an increased death rate, and this effect is independent of HIV viral load [21,125]. Whether infection and disease are simply markers of the immune dysfunction that follows HIV replication or whether HCMV promotes HIV progression is unknown [3]. Multiple mechanisms have been shown whereby HCMV (or other herpes viruses) could facilitate the pathogenicity of HIV [126], and some studies in haemophilia patients have supported a direct role for HCMV as a cofactor for HIV disease progression [127]. With the advent of HAART it is easy to discount the influence that HCMV has in the context of HIV infection since, to a large extent, HCMV-related diseases are now uncommon. However, it is worth noting two points. First, HAART is only widely available in the developed world and so HCMV and other opportunistic pathogens continue to substantially increase the morbidity and mortality of patients living with HIV in developing countries. Second, a recent study has indicated that even with successful control of HIV replication via HAART, the detection of transient HCMV replication by PCR is associated with an increased incidence of HIV disease progression and death [22]. Further research is required to define whether HCMV replication is just a marker of poor or sporadic immune reconstitution following HAART or is a direct accelerator of HIV pathogenesis.

Prevention and treatment of HCMV infection and disease

Prophylaxis and pre-emptive approaches for the prevention of the direct and indirect effects of HCMV

Globally, two modalities have been adopted for the prevention of HCMV disease in the setting of transplantation:

- prophylaxis, which is given to a patient population at risk of HCMV infection and disease (eg, D^+R^- solid organ transplant recipients) before there are any laboratory or clinical markers of active HCMV infection; and
- pre-emptive therapy, which is initiated as soon as possible after a specific laboratory marker of active HCMV infection becomes positive, indicative of future high-level replication and disease.

The rationale for the deployment of drugs to inhibit HCMV replication in both these modalities can be summarised using the threshold concept outlined on page 8. Therefore, by maintaining HCMV loads at very low levels using prophylaxis, the patient is prevented from moving into a viral load strata associated with a high risk of HCMV disease. In the case of a patient with high-level replication, pre-emptive therapy before the onset of symptoms will reduce their viral load and thus shift their probability of disease to a much lower level.

The period of prophylaxis usually matches the time frame at which the patient is most intensely immunosuppressed, and therefore at highest risk of HCMV infection and disease (ie, usually the first 100 days following transplant). Antiviral prophylaxis has been very successful at controlling HCMV infection, particularly in high-risk solid organ transplant patients, such as seronegative recipients of seropositive donor (D^+R^-) organs, reducing the incidence of HCMV disease by 50–70% [128]. In addition to inhibiting the direct effects of HCMV, prophylaxis with valaciclovir (in renal transplant recipients) and, more recently, ganciclovir (in liver transplant recipients) have been shown to reduce the incidence of acute rejection (*see* Figure 7.1) [129,130]. Prophylaxis has been

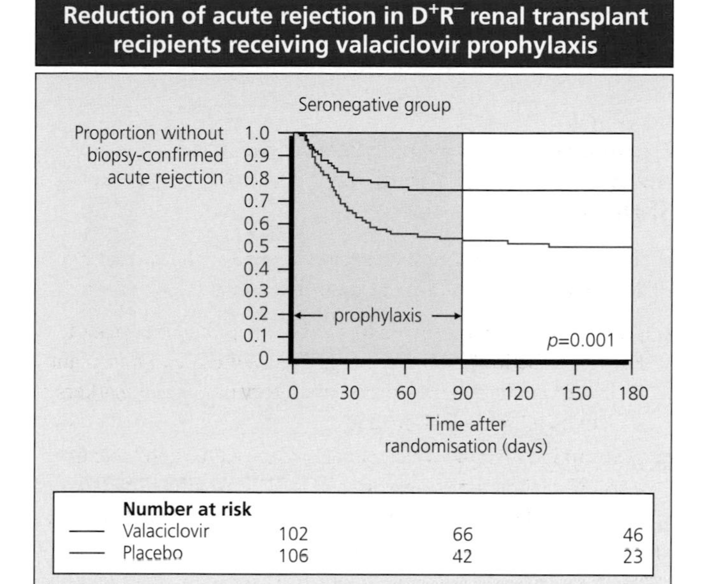

Figure 7.1. *D^+R^-, donor seropositive, recipient seronegative. Reproduced with permission from Lowance* et al *[129].*

shown to lower the risks of disease caused by herpes simplex virus or varicella-zoster virus, bacterial infections and protozoal infections (*see* Figure 7.2).

Prophylaxis prevents the development of HCMV disease in the majority of transplant recipients; however, this strategy leads to a shift in the time course of HCMV infection, with the occurrence of late-onset HCMV infection and disease several months after the transplantation [131]. The recent results of a trial comparing valganciclovir and oral ganciclovir prophylaxis (*see* Figures 7.3 and 7.4) following solid organ transplantation in D^+R^- high-risk patients aptly demonstrate this issue. The incidence of late HCMV infection and disease after cessation of prophylaxis is about 50% and 18%, respectively, illustrating the

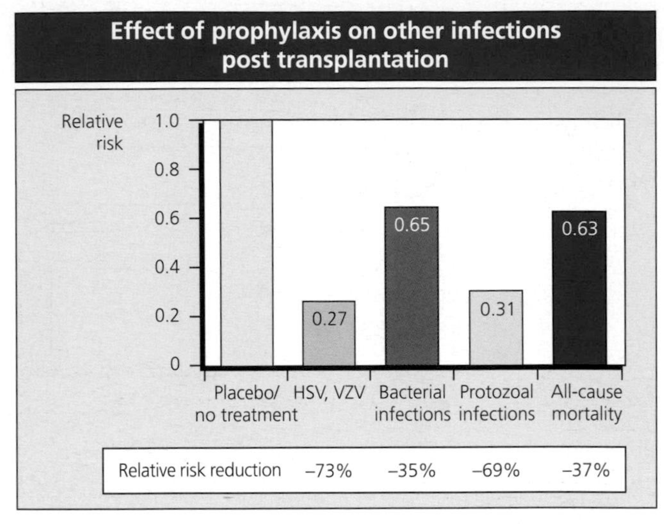

Figure 7.2. *HSV, herpes simplex virus; VZV, varicella-zoster virus. Data taken from Hodson* et al *[128].*

need for a strategy to be adopted to manage this late infection/disease appropriately. It should be remembered that the incidence of late HCMV disease observed in many prophylactic studies is substantially lower than the disease rates observed before the extensive deployment of antiviral chemotherapy for HCMV in the D^+R^- setting.

Pre-emptive therapy relies on the use of rapid, sensitive and reliable surveillance methods to diagnose HCMV replication at the earliest opportunity, thereby enabling therapy to be targeted to those at greatest risk of developing HCMV disease [133]. These laboratory methods include the HCMV pp65 antigenaemia assay and detection of HCMV DNA by PCR. Patients with evidence of high-level viral replication are eligible for pre-emptive therapy, which requires high doses of antiviral drugs aimed at quickly reducing viral replication. Treatment is administered to these patients in an attempt to prevent progression of asymptomatic infection into HCMV disease (viraemia can usually be identified several days before the onset of clinical symptoms). Pre-emptive

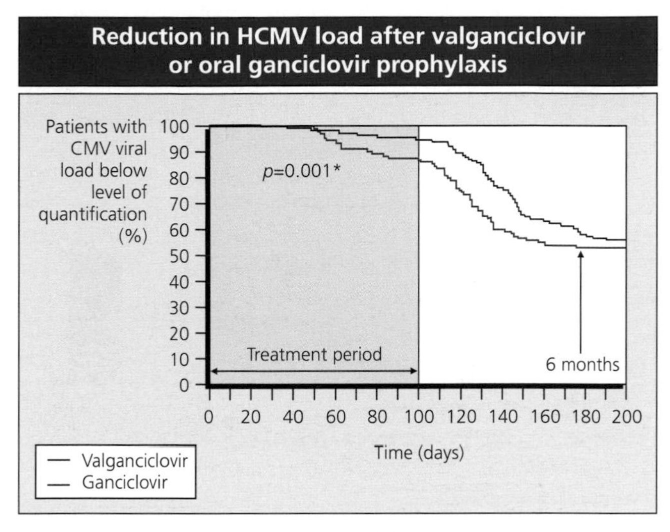

Figure 7.3. *Data taken from Paya* et al *[132].*

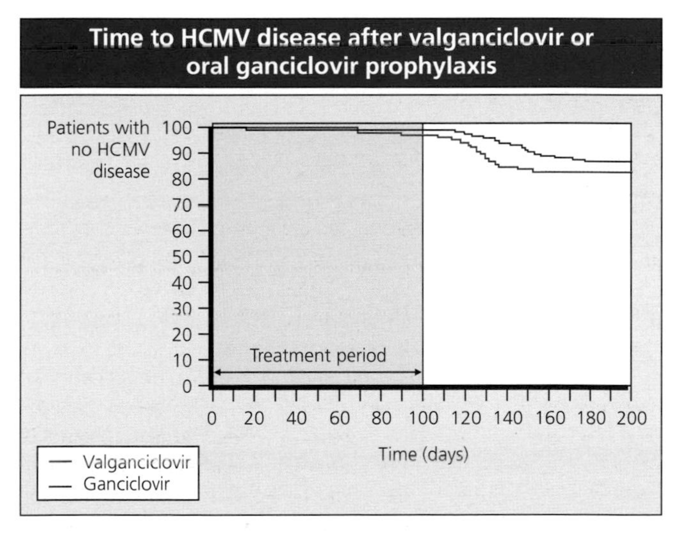

Figure 7.4. *Data taken from Paya* et al *[132].*

therapy has been suggested to offer some advantages for the management of HCMV infection [134], including reducing the number of patients exposed to potentially toxic antiviral therapy (which may result in less drug resistance) [17], and maximising cost–benefit. In addition, pre-emptive therapy enables limited replication of HCMV to occur, thus facilitating immune priming, which is likely to be important for future control of HCMV replication (this is in contrast to prophylaxis, which appears not to facilitate immune priming in the setting of stem cell transplantation) [50,134]. The success of pre-emptive strategies, however, requires:

- substantial commitment by the patient and their physician to regular monitoring for HCMV;
- excellent patient compliance;
- prompt assessment of samples by the laboratory; and
- implementation of treatment as soon as possible after detection of viral replication.

Furthermore, although PCR-guided pre-emptive treatment strategies have the potential advantage of very high sensitivity, which provides a high negative predictive value, the positive predictive value is variable and can be influenced by the analyte used [133]. It is also not clear whether the pre-emptive approach adequately addresses the indirect effects of HCMV (if not, prophylaxis aimed at both the direct and indirect effects of HCMV may be preferable) [6]. At present there is much debate about the relative merits of pre-emptive therapy versus prophylaxis in this setting [134,135]. It should be noted that between 25% and 33% of patients treated pre-emptively experience a second episode of DNAemia that requires further treatment.

The relative merits of prophylaxis and pre-emptive therapy have been extensively discussed elsewhere [134,135]. Nevertheless, there are key advantages and disadvantages to both approaches that are highlighted in Table 7.1.

Randomised controlled studies are clearly required to compare prophylaxis with pre-emptive therapy in terms of efficacy, evolution of drug resistance and appearance of late HCMV disease [5]. Nevertheless, it is likely that both clinical management strategies (prophylaxis and pre-emptive) provide an excellent way of minimising the impact of HCMV for an individual patient, although

The advantages and disadvantages to prophylaxis and pre-emptive therapy
Prophylaxis
Advantages • Universal or targeted • Eliminates direct and indirect effects of HCMV • Late infection/disease occurs when immunosuppressive therapy is less intensive
Disadvantages • Subset of patients remain at risk of late HCMV infection/disease after cessation of prophylaxis
Pre-emptive therapy
Advantages • Initiated based on virological markers • Minimises drug exposure
Disadvantages • Patients may require more than one treatment • May not eliminate the indirect effects of HCMV

Table 7.1. *Adapted from Emery [134] and Hart & Paya [135].*

the limitations and requirements of both approaches must be carefully considered. Indeed, it is likely that a mixed approach to patient management may be adopted whereby very high-risk patients receive prophylaxis while the lower-risk strata are managed pre-emptively. The current licensed indications for drugs used in the management of HCMV infections are summarised in Table 7.2. The valine ester forms of both aciclovir and ganciclovir allow substantial increases in bioavailabilty to be achieved over the parent aciclovir (67% versus 15%) and ganciclovir (60% versus 5%). The pharmacokinetic profile of this formulation of ganciclovir is shown in Figure 7.5.

The British Transplantation Society (BTS) recommendations for the prevention of HCMV disease through prophylaxis in solid organ transplant recipients are provided in Table 7.3 [137].

Licensed indications in the UK for drugs used to manage HCMV infection and disease

Drug	Description of action	Licensed indications
Valaciclovir	Valine ester of aciclovir with increased bioavailablity. Aciclovir is a cyclic nucleoside homologue of guanosine that is phosphorylated to its monophosphate form by the HCMV UL97 protein. It is active against HCMV in the triphosphate form where it acts as a chain terminator of viral DNA synthesis	Licensed for prophylaxis in renal transplant recipients
Valganciclovir	Valine ester of an acyclic nucleoside homologue of guanosine. Phosphorylated to its monophosphate form by the HCMV UL97 protein. The drug is active as the triphosphate moiety and acts as a chain terminator of viral DNA synthesis	Licensed for the treatment of HCMV retinitis in HIV-1-infected patients (900 mg bid). Licensed for maintenance therapy following treatment of HCMV retinitis in HIV-1-infected patients. Licensed for prevention of HCMV disease (prophylaxis 900 mg od) in high-risk ($D^{+}R^{-}$) solid organ transplant recipients
Ganciclovir (intravenous)	Acyclic nucleoside: homologue of guanosine. Phosphorylated to the monophosphate by HCMV UL97. Active as the triphosphate	Licensed for the treatment of life- or sight-threatening HCMV infections in immunocompromised hosts, including patients with AIDS, those undergoing iatrogenic immunosupression for organ transplantation or chemotherapy for neoplasias [128]
Cidofovir	Nucleotide monophosphate directly inhibiting HCMV DNA polymerase after phosphorylation by cell kinases to the triphosphate	Licensed in combination with probenecid for treatment of HCMV retinitis in AIDS patients where other agents are unsuitable

Table 7.2. *Continued opposite.*

Licensed indications in the UK for drugs used to manage HCMV infection and disease		
Drug	**Description of action**	**Comments**
Foscarnet	Inorganic pyrophosphate analogue directly inhibiting the HCMV DNA polymerase	Licensed for the treatment of HCMV retinitis in AIDS patients

Table 7.2. *(Continued).*

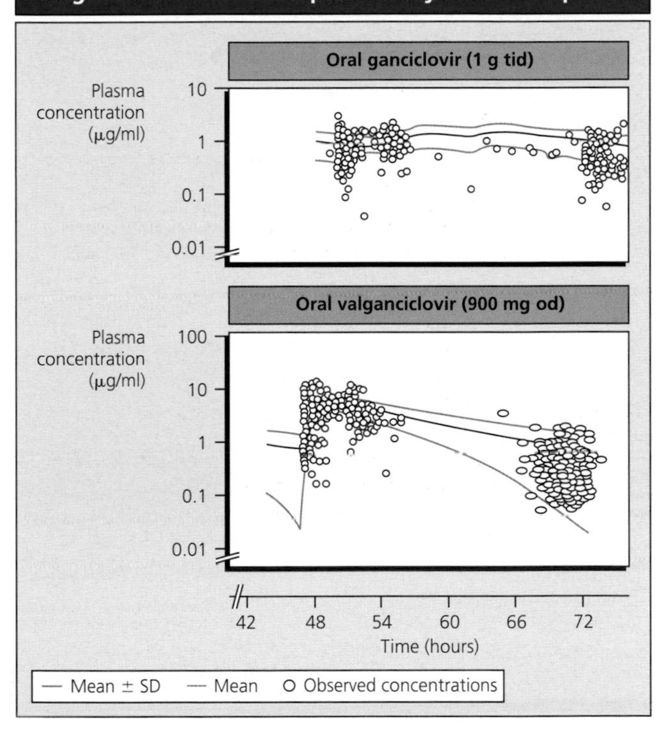

Figure 7.5. *A comparison of observed and model-predicted plasma levels of ganciclovir. SOT, solid organ transplant. Reproduced with permission from Wiltshire* et al *[136].*

Prophylaxis for prevention of HCMV disease in solid organ transplant recipients

Renal transplant recipients

In D^+/R^- patients:

- Valaciclovir for 90 days post transplant (Grade A)
- Oral ganciclovir for 90 days post transplant (Grade A)
- IV ganciclovir for 28 days (Grade A)
- Oral valganciclovir for 100 days (Grade A)
- High-dose oral aciclovir for 12 weeks (Grade B)
- Intermittent IV CMV-hyperimmune globulin for 12 weeks (Grade B)
- Serial measurements of viral load with treatment with IV ganciclovir or oral valganciclovir when levels predict disease (Grade B)
- Serial measurements of viral load with treatment with oral ganciclovir when levels predict disease (Grade A)

In D^+/R^+ patients*:

- No prophylaxis is recommended (Grade A)

Liver transplant recipients

In D^+/R^- patients:

- Oral ganciclovir for 90 days post transplant (Grade A)
- IV ganciclovir for 100 days (Grade A)
- Oral valganciclovir for 100 days (Grade A)
- Valaciclovir for 90 days post transplant (Grade C)
- Serial measurements of viral load with treatment with IV ganciclovir or oral valganciclovir when levels predict disease (Grade A)

In D^+/R^+ patients*:

- No prophylaxis is recommended (Grade A)

Kidney/pancreas transplant recipients

In D^+/R^- patients:

- Oral ganciclovir for 90 days post transplant (Grade C)
- IV ganciclovir for 28 days (Grade C)
- Oral valganciclovir for 100 days (Grade C)
- Valaciclovir for 90 days post transplant (Grade C)
- Serial measurements of viral load with treatment with IV ganciclovir when levels predict disease (Grade C)

In D^+/R^+ patients*:

- No prophylaxis is recommended (Grade C)

Table 7.3. *Continued opposite.*

Prophylaxis for prevention of HCMV disease in solid organ transplant recipients
Lung transplant recipients
In D^+/R^- patients: • Oral ganciclovir for 90 days post transplant (Grade B) • IV ganciclovir for 28 days then oral ganciclovir for 60 days (Grade B) • Valaciclovir for 90 days post transplant (Grade C) **In D^+/R^+ patients*:** • Oral ganciclovir for 90 days post transplant (Grade C) • IV ganciclovir for 28 days then oral ganciclovir for 60 days (Grade C) • Valaciclovir for 90 days post transplant (Grade C)
Heart transplant recipients
In D^+/R^- patients: • Oral valganciclovir for 100 days (Grade A) • Oral ganciclovir for 90 days post transplant (Grade B) • IV ganciclovir for 28 days (Grade B) • Valaciclovir for 90 days post transplant (Grade C) • Serial measurements of viral load with treatment with IV ganciclovir when levels predict disease (Grade C) **In D^+/R^+ patients*:** • No prophylaxis is recommended (Grade C)

Table 7.3. *(Continued). *Not receiving ATG/ALG/OKT3. D^+/R^+ patients receiving ATG/ALG/OKT3 should be treated following the recommendations of D^+/R^- patients. The British Transplantation Society (BTS) recommendations are graded using categories A to E, where A is the strongest recommendations in support of the treatment (based on high-quality studies); grade B recommendations are based upon cohort or other nonrandomised controlled studies; and grade C indicates that there is insufficient or contradictory evidence available. Guidelines are adapted from the BTS [137].*

Treatment of established HCMV disease

Although antiviral prophylaxis and pre-emptive therapy can be effective and successful, treatment of established (or full-blown clinical) HCMV disease is still required in patients who progress to symptoms. The advent of prophylaxis and pre-emptive therapeutic approaches in the transplant setting has substantially reduced the necessity to treat large numbers of patients with established disease, but inevitably there remains a subset who will require treatment despite the availability of such clinical management strategies. It should be noted that once HCMV disease is established, viral loads will be high, and a number of other sequalae of infection may have been initiated, not least by the host response to control replication. Consequently, the patient with established HCMV disease presents a very different clinical management scenario to one who is only experiencing asymptomatic DNAemia. Treatment strategies for established HCMV disease needs high efficacy of antiviral drugs that can quickly reduce the viral replication. Much of the data relating to treatment has been derived from HIV-1-infected patients presenting with sight-threatening HCMV retinitis. In some situations, such as HCMV pneumonitis, the addition of immunoglobulin may also be beneficial. In the past, antiviral drugs were administered for 2 weeks as standard, although increasingly therapy is now guided by the results of antigenaemia or PCR where evidence of control of viral replication indicates treatment duration.

Adoptive immunotherapy for HCMV

Since the seminal studies of Riddell and Greenberg [138] in Seattle in the early 1990s, there has been an increasing interest in using adoptive immunotherapy (infusion of T-cells able to control HCMV replication into patients), especially in the setting of stem cell transplantation. The advent of new technologies, such as class I HLA tetramers, and also different cell culture systems, including the use of dendritic cells, has enabled significant progress to be achieved [139–141]. Although no placebo-controlled study has been undertaken, a number of groups have shown that in stem cell recipients with persistent HCMV replication unresponsive to ganciclovir, the infusion of CD8/CD4 cells expanded against HCMV can lead to the effective control of replication. These studies illustrate the importance of CD4 T-cells in order to provide the appropriate help and chemokine environment for the HCMV-specific T-cells to survive and proliferate. Although this approach is not in routine use, a number of laboratories are investigating more cost-effective and efficient routes to generate HCMV-specific T-cells for adoptive immunotherapy.

Antiviral resistance

A potential drawback with the use of more aggressive immunosuppressive regimens coupled with more extensive antiviral therapy to control HCMV is increased incidence of drug-resistant strains of HCMV. Widespread and prolonged use of antiviral drugs in recipients after solid organ transplantation has changed the natural course of HCMV disease by delaying its onset, and a small subset of patients will experience active replication in the presence of low doses of antiviral agents (usually an environment that facilitates the development of drug-resistant strains of viruses) [5]. While we should not be complacent about the risk of development of drug-resistant strains of HCMV, there has been reassuring evidence from large clinical trials of ganciclovir in solid organ transplant recipients that drug resistance is not a significant problem in this patient population [142]. Similar data for short-term pre-emptive therapy in stem cell transplant recipients have also been published [143].

Historically, a high proportion (up to 71%) of HIV-infected patients with retinitis in the pre-HAART era, treated with intravenous ganciclovir for 3 weeks followed by long-term oral ganciclovir maintenance therapy, experienced genotypic drug-resistant HCMV [144]. In a recent trial of valganciclovir for induction and maintenance therapy of HCMV retinitis in AIDS patients, the incidence of drug resistance was 15% after 18 months [145]. This relatively high incidence of HCMV drug resistance in HIV-infected patients probably occurred for a number of reasons, including the extensive period of replication of HCMV that preceded the onset of retinitis (ie, drug-resistant mutants were likely to be present at low levels at the commencement of therapy) coupled with the low potency of oral ganciclovir at inhibiting replication of drug-resistant viruses [146] following a 3-week induction therapy with high-dose ganciclovir (5 mg/kg bid). Such a situation contrasts with the replication history of HCMV in the transplant setting (only a short period of high-level replication prior to therapeutic intervention) and the clinical management strategies that have been adopted.

However, ganciclovir-resistant HCMV infection can be a serious complication of solid organ transplantation and is associated with persistent viraemia, more frequent disease, more severe disease, a high rate of graft loss and high mortality [147–149]. There are a range of clinical scenarios associated with ganciclovir-resistance from asymptomatic viraemia to progressive tissue invasive disease with serious complications. The incidence of ganciclovir resistance in solid organ transplant patients receiving prophylaxis is estimated to be between 0% and 13% [147–149]. Resistance to ganciclovir appears to be a late post-transplant complication and is usually accounted for by mutations in the HCMV *UL97* gene, which codes for a viral protein kinase responsible for initial phosphorylation (and therefore activation) of ganciclovir (*see* Figure 7.6 and Table 7.2). Strains of HCMV that are resistant to ganciclovir through mutations within the *UL97* gene are less able to phosphorylate the drug. A number of genetic changes within the UL97 protein have been mapped and confirmed to confer drug resistance (*see* Figure 7.7). Less commonly, resistance to ganciclovir may be due to mutations in the HCMV *UL54* gene, which codes for HCMV DNA polymerase [4]. In the transplant population, ganciclovir resistance is predominantly seen in HCMV-seronegative recipients of organs from

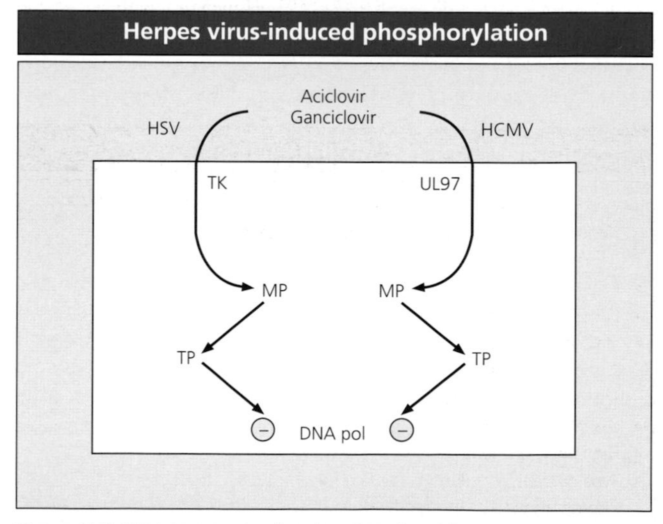

Figure 7.6. *HSV, herpes simplex virus; TK, thymidine kinase; MP, monophosphate; TP, triphosphate.*

Common mutations in the HCMV UL97 protein conferring ganciclovir resistance

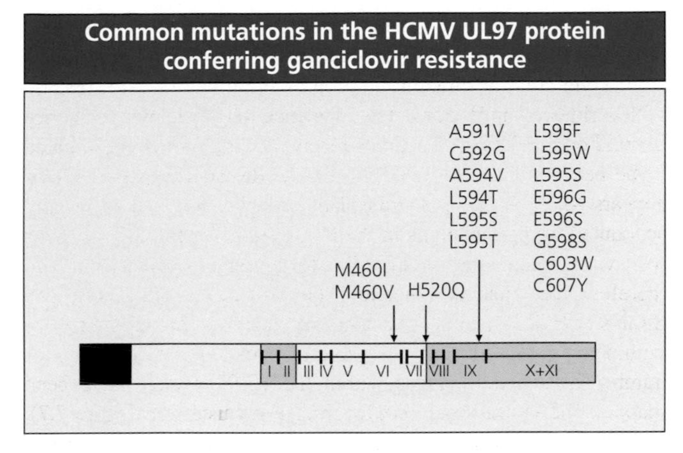

Figure 7.7.

seropositive donors, particularly those with potent immunosuppression and prolonged exposure to ganciclovir (especially oral ganciclovir) (*see* Table 7.4) [5,15,147–149]. However, analysis of the emergence of drug resistance in D^+R^- solid organ transplant

Factors associated with increased ganciclovir resistance

Factors that appear to be associated with increased drug resistance include:

- Donor seropositive/recipient seronegative status
- Primary infection
- Relapsing infection
- Suboptimal dose or duration of therapy
- Increased number of HCMV reactivations
- Prolonged exposure to ganciclovir
- Potent immunosuppression
- Use of antilymphocyte agents
- High peak viral loads
- Type of transplant (lung transplant patients appear to be disproportionately affected by drug resistance)

Table 7.4.

recipients randomised to receive valganciclovir (900 mg bid) prophylaxis for 100 days revealed that no cases of genotypic resistance were observed compared with 1.9% of cases in patients receiving oral ganciclovir (1 g tid) [142]. This observation is consistent with the increased drug potency against HCMV replication achieved with valganciclovir at the 900-mg once-daily dose over oral ganciclovir.

Among transplant recipients, lung transplant patients appear to be disproportionately affected by drug resistance [147], which may be because the level of immunosuppression in these patients is greater than in other transplant recipients. It has been observed that UL97 drug-resistant mutations are less fit than wild-type strains of HCMV so that in the absence of selection wild-type viruses repopulate at the expense of drug-resistant strains [146]. However, despite this observation, drug-resistant HCMV strains are fully able to cause disease and so cannot be ignored.

Other antiviral drugs that do not require intracellular phosphorylation to inhibit the viral DNA polymerase (eg, foscarnet and cidofovir) retain activity against most ganciclovir-resistant strains of HCMV and may be useful in managing drug-resistant disease [51]. Drug resistance against these agents map to the DNA polymerase only. In some cases, cross resistance and multidrug resistance within the DNA polymerase has been noted. At present, the development of antiviral resistance is uncommon in haematopoietic stem cell transplant patients, but mutants in both the HCMV DNA polymerase and the *UL97* gene have been reported [133].

8

Concluding remarks

HCMV is a remarkable virus in that it has evolved a range of genes that allow it to manipulate the environment of the human host so that it persists without major disease implications. However, when the delicate host–virus relationship is disturbed the virus becomes a major pathogenic force. In recent years, our understanding of HCMV pathogenesis and the function of many gene products has increased dramatically. These advances have been paralleled with the effective deployment of antiviral chemotherapy so that the devastating effects that HCMV disease once had in immunocompromised patients are now minimised. Consequently, we are now appreciating the more subtle effects that HCMV infection can have on the immunocompromised host and even in the immunocompetent individual. The future will continue to see a refinement in our understanding of HCMV and the development of newer approaches to control replication, including novel vaccines, new antiviral agents and the routine use of adoptive immunotherapy. It is certain that the lessons learned from the last 20 years of HCMV research and clinical management must not be ignored if we are to successfully control HCMV in the next 20 years.

References

1. Landolfo S, Gariglio M, Gribaudo G *et al.* **The human cytomegalovirus.** *Pharmacol Ther* 2003; **98**:269–297.

2. Dolan A, Cunningham C, Hector RD *et al.* **Genetic content of wild-type human cytomegalovirus.** *J Gen Virol* 2004; **85**:1301–1312.

3. Gandhi MK, Khanna R. **Human cytomegalovirus: clinical aspects, immune regulation, and emerging treatments.** *Lancet Infect Dis* 2004; **4**:725–738.

4. Anonymous. **Cytomegalovirus.** *Am J Transplant* 2004; **4**(Suppl 10):51–58.

5. Rowshani AT, Bemelman FJ, van Leeuwen EM *et al.* **Clinical and immunologic aspects of cytomegalovirus infection in solid organ transplant recipients.** *Transplantation* 2005; **79**:381–386.

6. Pereyra F, Rubin RH. **Prevention and treatment of cytomegalovirus infection in solid organ transplant recipients.** *Curr Opin Infect Dis* 2004; **17**:357–361.

7. Cope AV, Sabin C, Burroughs A *et al.* **Interrelationships among quantity of human cytomegalovirus (HCMV) DNA in blood, donor-recipient serostatus, and administration of methylprednisolone as risk factors for HCMV disease following liver transplantation.** *J Infect Dis* 1997; **176**:1484–1490.

8. Pusztai R, Lukacsi A, Kovacs I. **Mother-to-fetus transmission of cytomegalovirus. A review.** *Acta Microbiol Immunol Hung* 2004; **51**:385–401.

9. Grahame-Clarke C, Chan NN *et al.* **Human cytomegalovirus seropositivity is associated with impaired vascular function.** *Circulation* 2003; **108**:678–683.

10. Blum A, Giladi M, Weinberg M *et al.* **High anti-cytomegalovirus (CMV) IgG antibody titer is associated with coronary artery disease and may predict post-coronary balloon angioplasty restenosis.** *Am J Cardiol* 1998; **81**:866–868.

11. Zhou YF, Leon MB, Waclawiw MA *et al.* **Association between prior cytomegalovirus infection and the risk of restenosis after coronary atherectomy.** *N Engl J Med* 1996; **335**:624–630.

12. Stagno S, Reynolds DW, Tsiantos A. **Comparative serial virologic and serologic studies of symptomatic and subclinical congenitally and natally acquired cytomegalovirus infections.** *J Infect Dis* 1975; **132**:568–577.

13. Boppana SB, Fowler KB, Pass RF *et al.* **Congenital cytomegalovirus infection: association between virus burden in infancy and hearing loss.** *J Pediatr* 2005; **146**:817–823.

14. Emery VC, Sabin CA, Cope AV *et al.* **Application of viral-load kinetics to identify patients who develop cytomegalovirus disease after transplantation.** *Lancet* 2000; **355**:2032–2036.

15. Razonable RR, Emery VC; 11th Annual Meeting of the IHMF (International Herpes Management Forum). **Management of CMV infection and disease in transplant patients. 27–29 February 2004.** *Herpes* 2004; **11**:77–86.

16. Regoes RR, Bowen EF, Cope AV *et al.* **Modelling cytomegalovirus replication patterns in the human host: factors important for pathogenesis.** *Proc R Soc Lond B Biol Sci* 2006; 273:1961–1967.

17. Sagedal S, Hartmann A, Rollag H. **The impact of early cytomegalovirus infection and disease in renal transplant recipients.** *Clin Microbiol Infect* 2005; **11**:518–530.

18. Emery VC, Cope AV, Bowen EF *et al.* **The dynamics of human cytomegalovirus replication in vivo.** *J Exp Med* 1999; **190**:177–182.

19. Emery VC, Hassan-Walker AF, Burroughs AK *et al.* **Human cytomegalovirus (HCMV) replication dynamics in HCMV-naive and -experienced immunocompromised hosts**. *J Infect Dis* 2002; **185**:1723–1728.

20. Mattes FM, Hainsworth EG, Geretti AM *et al.* **A randomized, controlled trial comparing ganciclovir to ganciclovir plus foscarnet (each at half dose) for preemptive therapy of cytomegalovirus infection in transplant recipients.** *J Infect Dis* 2004; **189**:1355–1361.

21. Spector SA, Hsia K, Crager M *et al.* **Cytomegalovirus (CMV) DNA load is an independent predictor of CMV disease and survival in advanced AIDS.** *J Virol* 1999; **73**:7027–7030.

22. Deayton JR, Sabin CA, Johnson MA *et al.* **Importance of cytomegalovirus viraemia in risk of disease progression and death in HIV-infected patients receiving highly active antiretroviral therapy**. *Lancet* 2004; **363**:2116–2121.

23. Wohl DA, Zeng D, Stewart P *et al.* **Cytomegalovirus viremia, mortality, and end-organ disease among patients with AIDS receiving potent antiretroviral therapies.** *J Acquir Immune Defic Syndr* 2005; **38**:538–544.

24. Jabs DA, Gilpin AM, Min YI *et al.*; Studies of Ocular Complications of AIDS Research Group. **HIV and cytomegalovirus viral load and clinical outcomes in AIDS and cytomegalovirus retinitis patients: Monoclonal Antibody Cytomegalovirus Retinitis Trial.** *AIDS* 2002; **16**:877–887.

25. Danziger-Isakov LA, DelaMorena M, Hayashi RJ *et al.* **Cytomegalovirus viremia associated with death or retransplantation in pediatric lung-transplant recipients.** *Transplantation* 2003; **75**:1538–1543.

26. Gandhi MK, Wills MR, Sissons JG *et al.* **Human cytomegalovirus-specific immunity following haemopoietic stem cell transplantation.** *Blood Rev* 2003; **17**:259–264.

27. Compton T. **Receptors and immune sensors: the complex entry path of human cytomegalovirus.** *Trends Cell Biol* 2004; **14**:5–8.

28. Britt WJ, Boppana S. **Human cytomegalovirus virion proteins.** *Hum Immunol* 2004; **65**:395–402.

29. Boeckh M, Bowden RA, Storer B *et al.* **Randomized, placebo-controlled, double-blind study of a cytomegalovirus-specific monoclonal antibody (MSL-109) for prevention of cytomegalovirus infection after allogeneic hematopoietic stem cell transplantation.** *Biol Blood Marrow Transplant* 2001; **7**:343–351.

30. **MSL-109 adjuvant therapy for cytomegalovirus retinitis in patients with acquired immunodeficiency syndrome: the Monoclonal Antibody Cytomegalovirus Retinitis Trial. The Studies of Ocular Complications of AIDS Research Group. AIDS Clinical Trials Group.** *Arch Ophthalmol* 1997; **115**:1528–1536.

31. Jonjic S, Pavic I, Polic B *et al.* **Antibodies are not essential for the resolution of primary cytomegalovirus infection but limit dissemination of recurrent virus.** *J Exp Med* 1994; **179**:1713–1717.

32. Schleiss MR, Bourne N, Stroup G *et al.* **Protection against congenital cytomegalovirus infection and disease in guinea pigs, conferred by a purified recombinant glycoprotein B vaccine.** *J Infect Dis* 2004; **189**:1374–1381.

33. Chatterjee A, Harrison CJ, Britt WJ *et al.* **Modification of maternal and congenital cytomegalovirus infection by anti-glycoprotein b antibody transfer in guinea pigs.** *J Infect Dis* 2001; **183**:1547–1553.

34. Sylwester AW, Mitchell BL, Edgar JB *et al.* **Broadly targeted human cytomegalovirus-specific CD4+ and CD8+ T cells dominate the memory compartments of exposed subjects.** *J Exp Med* 2005; **202**:673–685.

35. Aubert G, Hassan-Walker AF, Madrigal JA *et al.* **Cytomegalovirus-specific cellular immune responses and viremia in recipients of allogeneic stem cell transplants.** *J Infect Dis* 2001; **184**:955–963.

36. Komatsu H, Sierro S, V Cuero A *et al.* **Population analysis of antiviral T cell responses using MHC class I-peptide tetramers.** *Clin Exp Immunol* 2003; **134**:9–12.

37. Appay V, Dunbar PR, Callan M *et al.* **Memory CD8+ T cells vary in differentiation phenotype in different persistent virus infections.** *Nat Med* 2002; **8**:379–385.

38. Wills MR, Carmichael AJ, Weekes MP *et al.* **Human virus-specific CD8+ CTL clones revert from CD45ROhigh to CD45RAhigh *in vivo*: CD45RAhighCD8+ T cells comprise both naive and memory cells.** *J Immunol* 1999; **162**:7080–7087.

39. Northfield J, Lucas M, Jones H *et al.* **Does memory improve with age? CD85j (ILT-2/LIR-1) expression on CD8 T cells correlates with 'memory inflation' in human cytomegalovirus infection.** *Immunol Cell Biol* 2005; **83**:182–188.

40. Akbar AN, Fletcher JM. **Memory T cell homeostasis and senescence during aging.** *Curr Opin Immunol* 2005; **17**:480–485.

41. Fletcher JM, Vukmanovic-Stejic M, Dunne PJ *et al.* **Cytomegalovirus-specific CD4+ T cells in healthy carriers are continuously driven to replicative exhaustion.** *J Immunol* 2005; **175**:8218–8225.

42. Gamadia LE, Rentenaar RJ, van Lier RA *et al.* **Properties of CD4(+) T cells in human cytomegalovirus infection.** *Hum Immunol* 2004; **65**:486–492.

43. Weekes MP, Wills MR, Sissons JG *et al.* **Long-term stable expanded human CD4+ T cell clones specific for human cytomegalovirus are distributed in both CD45RAhigh and CD45ROhigh populations.** *J Immunol* 2004; **173**:5843–5851.

44. Bronke C, Palmer NM, Jansen CA *et al.* **Dynamics of cytomegalovirus (CMV)-specific T cells in HIV-1-infected individuals progressing to AIDS with CMV end-organ disease.** *J Infect Dis* 2005; **191**:873–880.

45. Komanduri KV, Viswanathan MN, Wieder ED *et al.* **Restoration of cytomegalovirus-specific CD4+ T-lymphocyte responses after ganciclovir and highly active antiretroviral therapy in individuals infected with HIV-1.** *Nat Med* 1998; **4**:953–956.

46. Mocarski ES Jr. **Immune escape and exploitation strategies of cytomegaloviruses: impact on and imitation of the major histocompatibility system.** *Cell Microbiol* 2004; **6**:707–717.

47. Lilley BN, Ploegh HL. **Viral modulation of antigen presentation: manipulation of cellular targets in the ER and beyond.** *Immunol Rev* 2005; **207**:126–144.

48. Braud VM, Tomasec P, Wilkinson GW. **Viral evasion of natural killer cells during human cytomegalovirus infection.** *Curr Top Microbiol Immunol* 2002; **269**:117–129.

49. Gerna G, Baldanti R, evello MG. **Pathogenesis of human cytomegalovirus infection and cellular targets.** *Hum Immunol* 2004; **65**:381–386.

50. Das A. **Cytomegalovirus infection in solid organ transplantation. Economic implications.** *Pharmacoeconomics* 2003; **21**:467–475.

51. Kirubakaran SI. **Update: cytomegalovirus infection in HIV-infected patients – a review.** *Clin Microbiol Newsl* 2004; **26**:137–144.

52. Razonable RR, Brown RA, Wilson J *et al.* **The clinical use of various blood compartments for cytomegalovirus (CMV) DNA quantitation in transplant recipients with CMV disease.** *Transplantation* 2002; **73**:968–973.

53. Weinberg A, Schissel D, Giller R. **Molecular methods for cytomegalovirus surveillance in bone marrow transplant recipients.** *J Clin Microbiol* 2002; **40**:4203–4206.

54. Cortez KJ, Fischer SH, Fahle GA *et al.* **Clinical trial of quantitative real-time polymerase chain reaction for detection of cytomegalovirus in peripheral blood of allogeneic hematopoietic stem-cell transplant recipients.** *J Infect Dis* 2003; **188**:967–972.

55. Mengelle C, Sandres-Saune K, Pasquier C *et al.* **Automated extraction and quantification of human cytomegalovirus DNA in whole blood by real-time PCR assay.** *J Clin Microbiol* 2003; **41**:3840–3845.

56. Barbi M, Binda S, Primache V *et al.* **Cytomegalovirus DNA detection in Guthrie cards: a powerful tool for diagnosing congenital infection.** *J Clin Virol* 2000; **17**:159–165.

57. Binda S, Caroppo S, Dido P *et al.* **Modification of CMV DNA detection from dried blood spots for diagnosing congenital CMV infection**. *J Clin Virol* 2004; **30**:276–279.

58. van der Knaap MS, Vermeulen G, Barkhof F *et al.* **Pattern of white matter abnormalities at MR imaging: use of polymerase chain reaction testing of Guthrie cards to link pattern with congenital cytomegalovirus infection.** *Radiology* 2004; **230**:529–536.

59. Revello MG, Zavattoni M, Sarasini A *et al.* **Human cytomegalovirus in blood of immunocompetent persons during primary infection: prognostic implications for pregnancy.** *J Infect Dis* 1998; **177**:1170–1175.

60. Lazzarotto T, Gabrielli L, Lanari M *et al.* **Congenital cytomegalovirus infection: recent advances in the diagnosis of maternal infection.** *Hum Immunol* 2004; **65**:410–415.

61. Riegler S, Hebart H, Einsele H *et al.* **Monocyte-derived dendritic cells are permissive to the complete replicative cycle of human cytomegalovirus.** *J Gen Virol* 2000; **81**:393–399.

62. Sinzger C, Grefte A, Plachter B *et al.* **Fibroblasts, epithelial cells, endothelial cells and smooth muscle cells are major targets of human cytomegalovirus infection in lung and gastrointestinal tissues.** *J Gen Virol* 1995; **76**:741–750.

63. Schrier RD, Nelson JA, Oldstone MB. **Detection of human cytomegalovirus in peripheral blood lymphocytes in a natural infection.** *Science* 1985; **230**:1048–1051.

64. Plachter B, Sinzger C, Jahn G. **Cell types involved in replication and distribution of HCMV.** *Adv Virus Res* 1996; **46**:195–261.

65. Kondo K, Kaneshima H, Mocarski ES. **Human cytomegalovirus latent infection of granulocyte-macrophage progenitors.** *Proc Natl Acad Sci USA* 1994; **91**:11879–11883.

66. Castillo JP, Kowalik TF. **HCMV infection: modulating the cell cycle and cell death.** *Int Rev Immunol* 2004; **23**:113–139.

67. Revello MG, Gerna G. **Diagnosis and management of human cytomegalovirus infection in the mother, fetus and newborn infant.** *Clin Microbiol Rev* 2002; **15**:680–715.

68. Sissons JG, Carmichael AJ. **Clinical aspects and management of cytomegalovirus infection.** *J Infect* 2002; **44**:78–83.

69. Griffiths PD. **Cytomegalovirus.** In: *Principles and Practice of Clinical Virology, Fourth Edition.* Edited by Zuckerman AJ, Banatrala JE, Pattison JR. John Wiley & Sons, 2002.

70. Burny W, Liesnard C, Donner C *et al.* **Epidemiology, pathogenesis and prevention of congenital cytomegalovirus infection.** *Expert Rev Anti Infect Ther* 2004; **2**:881–894.

71. Fowler KB, Stagno S, Pass RF. **Maternal immunity and prevention of congenital cytomegalovirus infection.** *JAMA* 2003; **289**:1008–1011.

72. National Center for Infectious Diseases. **Cytomegalovirus (CMV) infection.** Available at: *www.cdc.gov/ncidod/diseases/cmv.htm.*

73. Stagno S, Pass RF, Cloud G *et al.* **Primary cytomegalovirus infection in pregnancy. Incidence, transmission to fetus, and clinical outcome.** *JAMA* 1986; **256**:1904–1908.

74. Griffiths PD, Walter S. **Cytomegalovirus.** *Curr Opin Infect Dis* 2005; **18**:241–245.

75. Fowler KB, Stagno S, Pass RF *et al.* **The outcome of congenital cytomegalovirus infection in relation to maternal antibody status.** *N Engl J Med* 1992; **326**:663–667.

76. Saigal S, Lunyk O, Larke RP *et al.* **The outcome in children with congenital cytomegalovirus infection. A longitudinal follow-up study.** *Am J Dis Child* 1982; **136**:896–901.

77. Williamson WD, Demmler GJ, Percy AK *et al.* **Progressive hearing loss in infants with asymptomatic congenital cytomegalovirus infection.** *Pediatrics* 1992; **90**:862–866.

78. Fowler KB, McCollister FP, Dahle AJ *et al.* **Progressive and fluctuating sensorineural hearing loss in children with asymptomatic congenital cytomegalovirus infection.** *J Pediatr* 1997; **130**:624–630.

79. Dahle AJ, Fowler KB, Wright JD *et al.* **Longitudinal investigation of hearing disorders in children with congenital cytomegalovirus.** *J Am Acad Audiol* 2000; **11**:283–290.

80. Lazzarotto T, Guerra B, Spezzacatena P *et al.* **Prenatal diagnosis of congenital cytomegalovirus infection.** *J Clin Microbiol* 1998; **36**:3540–3544.

81. Lazzarotto T, Gabrielli L, Foschini MP *et al.* **Congenital cytomegalovirus infection in twin pregnancies: viral load in the amniotic fluid and pregnancy outcome.** *Pediatrics* 2003; **112**:e153–e157.

82. Hamprecht K, Maschmann J, Vochem M *et al.* **Epidemiology of transmission of cytomegalovirus from mother to preterm infant by breastfeeding.** *Lancet* 2001; **357**:513–518.

83. Yeager AS, Palumbo PE, Malachowski N *et al.* **Sequelae of maternally derived cytomegalovirus infections in premature infants.** *J Pediatr* 1983; **102**:918–922.

84. Rubin RH. **The indirect effects of cytomegalovirus infection on the outcome of organ transplantation.** *JAMA* 1989; **261**:3607–3609.

85. Llungman P, Griffiths P, Paya C. **Definitions of cytomegalovirus infection and disease in transplant recipients.** *Clin Infect Dis* 2002; **34**:1094–1907.

86. Paya CV, Wilson JA, Espy MJ *et al.* **Preemptive use of oral ganciclovir to prevent cytomegalovirus infection in liver transplant patients: a randomized, placebo-controlled trial.** *J Infect Dis* 2002; **185**.854–860.

87. Patel R, Paya CV. **Infections in solid-organ transplant recipients.** *Clin Microbiol Rev* 1997; **10**:86–124.

88. Sia IG, Patel R. **New strategies for prevention and therapy of cytomegalovirus infection and disease in solid-organ transplant recipients.** *Clin Microbiol Rev* 2000; **13**:83–121.

89. Pour-Reza-Gholi F, Labibi A, Farrokhi F *et al.* **Signs and symptoms of cytomegalovirus disease in kidney transplant recipients.** *Transplant Proc* 2005; **37**:3056–3058.

90. Drew WL. **Cytomegalovirus infection in patients with AIDS.** *Clin Infect Dis* 1992; **14**:608–615.

91. Kahraman G, Krepler K, Franz C *et al.* **Seven years of HAART impact on ophthalmic management of HIV-infected patients.** *Ocul Immunol Inflamm* 2005; **13**:213–218.

92. Deayton JR, Sabin CA, Britt WB *et al.* **Rapid reconstitution of humoral immunity against cytomegalovirus but not HIV following highly active antiretroviral therapy.** *AIDS* 2002; **16**:2129–2135.

93. Deayton J, Mocroft A, Wilson P *et al.* **Loss of cytomegalovirus (CMV) viraemia following highly active antiretroviral therapy in the absence of specific anti-CMV therapy.** *AIDS* 1999; **13**:1203–1206.

94. Nordoy I, Muller F, Nordal KP *et al.* **The role of the tumor necrosis factor system and interleukin-10 during cytomegalovirus infection in renal transp recipients.** *J Infect Dis* 2000; **181**:51–57.

95. Durandy A. **Anti-B cell and anti-cytokine therapy for the treatmen transplant lymphoproliferative disorder: past, present, and future.** *T Dis* 2001; **3**:104–107.

96. Fishman JA, Rubin RH. **Infection in organ-transplant recipients.** *N Engl J Med* 1998; **338**:1741–1751.

97. Ison MG, Fishman JA. **Cytomegalovirus pneumonia in transplant recipients.** *Clin Chest Med* 2005; **26**:691–705.

98. Griffiths PD. **The 2001 Garrod lecture. The treatment of cytomegalovirus infection.** *J Antimicrob Chemother* 2002; **49**:243–253.

99. Kotton CN, Fishman JA. **Viral infection in the renal transplant recipient.** *J Am Soc Nephrol* 2005; **16**:1758–1774.

100. Paya CV. **Indirect effects of CMV in the solid organ transplant patient.** *Transpl Infect Dis* 1999; **1**(Suppl 1):8–12.

101. Rubin RH. **Impact of cytomegalovirus infection on organ transplant recipients.** *Rev Infect Dis* 1990; **12**(Suppl 7):S754–S766.

102. Ho M. **Cytomegalovirus infection and indirect sequelae in the immunocompromised transplant patient.** *Transplant Proc* 1991; **23**(Suppl 1):2–7.

103. Chatterjee SN, Fiala M, Weiner J *et al.* **Primary cytomegalovirus and opportunistic infections: incidence in renal transplant recipients.** *JAMA* 1978; **240**:2446–2449.

104. Cainelli F, Vento S. **Infections and solid organ transplant rejection: a cause-and-effect relationship?** *Lancet Infect Dis* 2002; **2**:539–549.

105. Gamadia LE, Remmerswaal EB, Surachno S *et al.* **Cross-reactivity of cytomegalovirus-specific CD8+ T cells to allo-major histocompatibility complex class I molecules.** *Transplantation* 2004; **77**:1879–1885.

106. Gupta P, Hart J, Cronin D *et al.* **Risk factors for chronic rejection after pediatric liver transplantation.** *Transplantation* 2001; **72**:1098–1102.

107. Tolkhoff-Rubin NE, Fishman JA *et al.* **The bidirectional relationship between cytomegalovirus and allograft injury.** *Transplant Proc* 2001; **33**:1773–1775.

108. Zamora MR. **Cytomegalovirus and lung transplantation.** *Am J Transplant* 2004; **4**:1219–1226.

109. von Willebrand E, Pettersson E, Ahonen J *et al.* **CMV infection, class II antigen expression, and human kidney allograft rejection.** *Transplantation* 1986; **42**:364–367.

110. Ustinov JA, Loginov RJ, Bruggeman CA *et al.* **Cytomegalovirus induces class II expression in rat heart endothelial cells.** *J Heart Lung Transplant* 1993; **12**:644–651.

111. Kloover JS, Soots AP, Krogerus LA *et al.* **Rat cytomegalovirus infection in kidney allograft recipients is associated with increased expression of intracellular adhesion molecule-1 vascular adhesion molecule-1, and their ligands leukocyte function antigen-1 and very late antigen-4 in the graft.** *Transplantation* 2000; **9**:2641–2647.

Koskinen PK. **The association of the induction of vascular cell adhesion ule-1 with cytomegalovirus antigenemia in human heart allografts.** *tation* 1993; **56**:1103–1108.

n A, Mege JL, Reynaud M *et al.* **Monitoring of alveolar macrophage tumor necrosis factor-alpha and interleukin-6 in lung transplant**

recipients. Marseille and Montreal Lung Transplantation Group. *Am J Respir Crit Care Med* 1994; **150**:684–689.

114. Toyoda M, Galfayan K, Galera OA *et al.* **Cytomegalovirus infection induces anti-endothelial cell antibodies in cardiac and renal allograft recipients.** *Transpl Immunol* 1997; **5**:104–111.

115. Hjelmesaeth J, Sagedal S, Hartmann A *et al.* **Asymptomatic cytomegalovirus infection is associated with increased risk of new-onset diabetes mellitus and impaired insulin release after renal transplantation.** *Diabetologia* 2004; **47**:1550–1156.

116. Paya CV. **Prevention of cytomegalovirus disease in recipients of solid-organ transplants.** *Clin Infect Dis* 2001; **32**:596–603.

117. Kol A, Libby P. **The mechanisms by which infectious agents may contribute to atherosclerosis and its clinical manifestations.** *Trends Cardiovasc Med* 1998; [illegible]:191–199.

118. Boeckh M, Nichols WG, Papanicolaou G *et al.* **Cytomegalovirus in hemato-[illegible]tic stem cell transplant recipients: Current status, known challenges, and [illegible]e strategies.** *Biol Blood Marrow Transplant* 2003; **9**:543–558.

119. Boeckh M, Fries B, Nichols WG. **Recent advances in the prevention of CMV infection and disease after hematopoietic stem cell transplantation.** *Pediatr Transplant* 2004; **8**(Suppl 5):19–27.

120. Boeckh M, Nichols WG. **The impact of cytomegalovirus serostatus of donor and recipient before hematopoietic stem cell transplantation in the era of anti-viral prophylaxis and preemptive therapy.** *Blood* 2004; **103**:2003–2008.

121. Nichols WG, Corey L, Gooley T *et al.* **High risk of death due to bacterial and fungal infection among cytomegalovirus (CMV)-seronegative recipients of stem cell transplants from seropositive donors: evidence for indirect effects of primary CMV infection.** *J Infect Dis* 2002; **185**:273–282.

122. Soderberg C, Larsson S, Rozell BL *et al.* **Cytomegalovirus-induced CD13-specific autoimmunity—a possible cause of chronic graft-vs-host disease.** *Transplantation* 1996; **61**:600–609.

123. Hernandez-Boluda JC, Lis MJ, Goterris R *et al.* **Guillain-Barre syndrome associated with cytomegalovirus infection after allogeneic hematopoietic stem cell transplantation.** *Transpl Infect Dis* 2005; **7**:93–96.

124. Reddy V, Meier-Kriesche HU, Greene S *et al.* **Increased levels of tumor necrosis factor alpha are associated with an increased risk of cytomegalovirus infection after allogeneic hematopoietic stem cell transplantation.** *Biol Blood Marrow Transplant* 2005; **11**:698–705.

125. Bowen EF, Wilson P, Cope A *et al.* **Cytomegalovirus retinitis in AIDS patients: influence of cytomegaloviral load on response to ganciclovir, time to recurrence and survival.** *AIDS* 1996; **10**:1515–1520.

126. Griffiths PD. **Studies to further define viral co-factors for human immunodeficiency virus.** *J Gen Virol* 1998; **79**:213–220.

127. Webster A, Lee CA, Cook DG *et al.* **Cytomegalovirus infection and progression towards AIDS in haemophiliacs with human immunodeficiency virus infection.** *Lancet* 1989; **2**:63–66.

128. Hodson Em, Jones CA, Webster AC *et al.* **Antiviral medications to prevent cytomegalovirus disease and early death in recipients of solid-organ transplants: a systematic review of ransomised controlled trials.** *Lancet* 2005; **365**:2105–2215.

129. Lowance D, Neumayer HH, Legendre CM *et al.* **Valacyclovir for the prevention of cytomegalovirus disease after renal transplantation. International Valacyclovir Cytomegalovirus Prophylaxis Transplantation Study Group.** *N Engl J Med* 1999; **340**:1462–1470.

130. Slifkin M, Ruthazer R, Freeman R *et al.* **Impact of cytomegalovirus prophylaxis on rejection following orthotopic liver transplantation.** *Liver Transpl* 2005; **11**:1597–1602.

131. Hebart H, Einsele H. **Clinical aspects of CMV infection after stem cell transplantation.** *Hum Immunol* 2004; **65**:432–436.

132. Paya C, Humar A, Dominguez E *et al.* **Efficacy and safety of valganciclovir vs oral ganciclovir for prevention of cytomegalovirus disease in solid organ tran plant recipients.** *Am J Transplant* 2004; **4**:611–620.

133. Peggs KS, Mackinnon S. **Cytomegalovirus: the role of CMV p haematopoietic stem cell transplantation.** *Int J Biochem Cell Biol* 20 **36**:695–701.

134. Emery VC. **Prophylaxis for CMV should not now replace pre-emptive therapy in solid organ transplantation.** *Rev Med Virol* 2001; **11**:83–86.

135. Hart GD, Paya CV. **Prophylaxis for CMV should now replace pre-emptive therapy in solid organ transplantation.** *Rev Med Virol* 2001; **11**:73–81.

136. Wiltshire H, Hirankarn S, Farrell C *et al*;Valganciclovir Solid Organ Transplant Study Group. **Pharmacokinetic profile of ganciclovir after its oral administration and from its prodrug, valganciclovir, in solid organ transplant recipients.** *Clin Pharmacokinet* 2005; **44**:495–507.

137. British Transplantation Society. *Guidelines for the Prevention and Management of Cytomegalovirus Disease after Solid Organ Transplantation. 2nd edition.* London: British Transplantation Society, 2004.

138. Walter EA, Greenberg PD, Gilbert MJ *et al.* **Reconstitution of cellular immunity against cytomegalovirus in recipients of allogeneic bone marrow by transfer of T-cell clones from the donor.** *N Engl J Med* 1995; **333**:1038–1044.

139. Peggs KS, Mackinnon S. **Augmentation of virus-specific immunity after hematopoietic stem cell transplantation by adoptive T-cell therapy.** *Hum Immunol* 2004; **65**:550–557.

140. Einsele H, Roosnek E, Rufer N *et al.* **Infusion of cytomegalovirus (CMV)-specific T cells for the treatment of CMV infection not responding to antiviral chemotherapy.** *Blood* 2002; **99**:3916–3922.

141. Cobbold M, Khan N, Pourgheysari B *et al.* **Adoptive transfer of cytomegalovirus-specific CTL to stem cell transplant patients after selection by HLA-peptide tetramers.** *J Exp Med* 2005; **202**:379–386.

142. Boivin G, Goyette N, Gilbert C *et al.* **Absence of cytomegalovirus-resistance mutations after valganciclovir prophylaxis, in a prospective multicenter study of lid-organ transplant recipients.** *J Infect Dis* 2004; **189**:1615–1618.

143. Gilbert C, Roy J, Belanger R *et al.* **Lack of emergence of cytomegalovirus UL97 mutations conferring ganciclovir (GCV) resistance following preemptive GCV therapy in allogeneic stem cell transplant recipients.** *Antimicrob Agents Chemother* 2001; **45**:3669–3671.

144. Bowen EF, Emery VC, Wilson P *et al.* **Cytomegalovirus polymerase chain reaction viraemia in patients receiving ganciclovir maintenance therapy for retinitis.** *AIDS* 1998; **12**:605–611.

145. Boivin G, Gilbert C, Gaudreau A *et al.* **Rate of emergence of cytomegalovirus (CMV) mutations in leukocytes of patients with acquired immunodeficiency syndrome who are receiving valganciclovir as induction and maintenance therapy for CMV retinitis.** *J Infect Dis* 2001; **184**:1598–1602.

146. Emery VC, Griffiths PD. **Prediction of cytomegalovirus load and resistance patterns after antiviral chemotherapy.** *Proc Natl Acad Sci USA* 2000; **97**:8039–8044.

147. Limaye AP, Corey L, Koelle DM *et al.* **Emergence of ganciclovir-resistant [illegible]omegalovirus disease among recipients of solid-organ transplants.** *Lancet* [illegible]); **356**:645–649.

[illegible] Limaye AP. **Ganciclovir-resistant cytomegalovirus in organ transplant recip-[illegible]nts.** *Clin Infect Dis* 2002; **35**:866–872.

149. Kruger RM, Shannon WD, Arens MQ *et al.* **The impact of ganciclovir-resistant cytomegalovirus infection after lung transplantation.** *Transplantation* 1999; **68**:1272–1279.